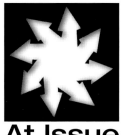

At Issue

COVID-19 and
Other Pandemics

Other Books in the At Issue Series

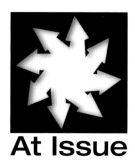

At Issue

COVID-19 and Other Pandemics

Barbara Krasner, Book Editor

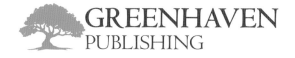

GREENHAVEN
PUBLISHING

Published in 2022 by Greenhaven Publishing, LLC
353 3rd Avenue, Suite 255, New York, NY 10010

Copyright © 2022 by Greenhaven Publishing, LLC

First Edition

Articles in Greenhaven Publishing anthologies are often edited for length to meet page
requirements. In addition, original titles of these works are changed to clearly present
the main thesis and to explicitly indicate the author's opinion. Every effort is made to
ensure that Greenhaven Publishing accurately reflects the original intent of the authors.
Every effort has been made to trace the owners of the copyrighted material.

Cover image: Mongkolchon Akesin/Shutterstock

Library of Congress Cataloging-in-Publication Data

Names: Krasner, Barbara, editor.
Title: COVID-19 and other pandemics / Barbara Krasner, book editor.
Description: First edition. | New York : Greenhaven Publishing, 2022. |
  Series: At issue | Includes bibliographical references and index. |
  Summary: "From the Black Death of the fourteenth century to HIV/AIDS
  and the recent COVID-19 crisis, pandemics and disease
  outbreaks have devastated societies, wiped out significant portions of
  populations, and necessitated political, social, and scientific changes
  to address these public health catastrophes. What have scientists and
  policymakers learned from historical pandemics, and what can be done to
  prevent future outbreaks? Journalists, politicians, medical
  professionals, and other experts from a range of fields weigh in on how
  pandemics happen and potential means of controlling them"-- Provided by
  publisher.
Identifiers: LCCN 2019056537 | ISBN 9781534507302 (library binding) | ISBN
  9781534507296 (paperback) | 9781534507319 (ebook)
Subjects: LCSH: Epidemics--Juvenile literature.
Classification: LCC RA653.5 .P38 2022 | DDC 614.4--dc23
LC record available at https://lccn.loc.gov/2019056537

Manufactured in the United States of America

Website: http://greenhavenpublishing.com

Contents

Introduction

I n 2020, a new and deadly virus ravaged the world and changed our lives forever. People were confined to their homes. Economies were severely impacted. Office buildings, schools, restaurants, gyms, museums, movie theaters, and other places that attract large groups of people closed down in order to stop the spread. Within one year of the official declaration of COVID-19's classification as a pandemic (a pandemic is the spread of infectious disease throughout the world), there were over 118 million cases, and more than 2.6 million people were dead from the virus or complications from it.[1] Virtually no one on the planet was unaffected by this disease.

To find a comparable event, you would have to go back in history almost exactly 100 years ago to the influenza pandemic of 1918–19. Some called it the Spanish flu. This virus killed an estimated 50 to 100 million people.[2] It caused more deaths than World War I.

But influenza was not the first major outbreak of cataclysmic disease. In the sixth century CE, a plague struck an Egyptian port. At first, those affected suffered from bloody noses. But then they developed swollen lymph nodes under their arms, on their neck, or in the groin. Black pustules eventually covered their body. The outbreak became known as the bubonic plague, and after about nine years it penetrated the city of Constantinople, the capital of the Eastern Roman Empire. Thousands of people died each day, and ships carried corpses out to sea. No remedies were available. The plague finally lost its impact after about one hundred years. No one knew what exactly had brought it on or when it would terrorize the population again.[3]

It reappeared in the fourteenth century, traveling along trade routes from China across the Black Sea into Europe. This pandemic—known as the Black Death—lasted from 1347 to

1351 and decimated the population. The Mongols used the plague as a biological weapon, tossing affected bodies over city walls to advance their conquest. About one-fifth of the world's population died as a result. With many of the people now gone, everyday life changed: Wars stopped, trade stopped, and there were fewer people to farm and to receive an education. But now that there was more food, people began to live longer.[4]

Throughout history, pandemics and outbreaks of deadly infectious diseases have delivered some positive outcomes amidst the devastation. Biologically, the human immune system can strengthen as a result. Environmentally, pandemics like the Black Death have served as a wake-up call for improved sanitary conditions and personal hygiene practices. Medically, research into these diseases—most notably influenza—has led to practices such as washing hands, and sustained medical research has isolated and identified the causes of these diseases and formulated revolutionary treatments such as antibiotics and vaccines. Socially, the Black Death led to a decrease in the political power of the church and, some experts say, the end of the feudal system.[5]

Pandemics and outbreaks tested everyday beliefs. For example, many supposed the Black Death was a religious warning that affected only sinners. The yellow fever epidemic in late eighteenth-century America affected how African Americans and slaves were treated, because many believed they were immune to this disease. However, this belief also contributed to racial prejudices.[6]

It is difficult to harness a moving target. New strains and mutations of diseases emerge, rendering previous remedies and preventative measures ineffective. Antibiotic resistance is one issue related to this. Vaccinations, too, may fight against one strain but not another. In recent years, some social and religious groups have publicly voiced opposition to vaccinations, instigating debates about their use and whether they should be mandated. Social media sparks the debates and allows misinformation to proliferate and sway public opinion in harmful directions.

Fear of widespread infectious disease can sway governmental actions as well. For instance, in 1976, US president Gerald Ford mounted an immunization campaign against the swine flu. Some older people recalled the terror of the 1918 flu pandemic and their fear spread to younger generations. More than forty million Americans received vaccines to protect them from the swine flu. However, the disease remained isolated. It affected only a handful of people and caused only one death.[7]

Although some researchers claim it is better to have a vaccination without an epidemic than an epidemic without a vaccine, new problems with vaccinations can emerge. In the case of the 1976 swine flu, the maker of the flu vaccine confused its viruses, and consequently its vaccine was formulated to treat a different strain. More than 500 people had a serious reaction to a vaccine that had been developed earlier in the year, and 23 people died from the vaccine. The vaccine to fight COVID-19 was developed and rolled out in record time, instilling hope in people around the world for a return to normalcy. Still, some resisted vaccination because of an outright distrust of the government. On the other hand, vaccines have effectively controlled or eradicated many diseases, including polio, smallpox, diphtheria, tetanus, yellow fever, whooping cough, and measles.

Technology can play an important role in controlling pandemics and outbreaks. Digital platforms, advanced analytics, and machine learning algorithms can be used to protect those at risk, such as babies against diseases like measles. Still, as important as diagnostic and surveillance tools are, poverty-stricken areas tend to lack them. Outbreak incidents may go unnoticed and unreported in these areas. Statistics are often a matter of debate as well, as they are difficult to gather, particularly in poor areas.

The decline in HIV infection rates and AIDS-related deaths points to the efficacy of various preventative measures and treatments. These include HIV testing, pre-exposure prophylaxis to prevent those at high risk of contracting HIV from becoming infected, education for at-risk populations on how to prevent transmission (such as through the use of condoms and not sharing intravenous needles), and the potential development of an HIV vaccine. However, people still contract HIV/AIDS despite these efforts, and lower-income countries are disproportionately impacted with less access to treatment and preventative medicine.[8]

People look to policymakers for responses to stop outbreaks from spreading and to prevent future occurrences. Cases of Ebola that broke out in West Africa are an example of this. In the 2014–2015 outbreak, the United States played a major role in responding, but it has been less involved recently.[9] Funding and other forms of support from other nations and the World Health Organization are considered necessary to address the outbreak in low-income areas. The US has also responded with travel bans, though this is a source of controversy. Countries with high rates of transmission create policies to better educate the public about hygiene, disinfection, and prevention, though improved health infrastructure is also considered necessary. However, this may not be possible to achieve without international support.

The severe acute respiratory syndrome (SARS) outbreak in 2003 provided evidence that domestic governmental policies have an important effect on the spread of diseases across international boundaries.[10] Before the COVID-19 outbreak, the possible mutation of the H5N1 avian flu virus was a primary concern of scientists, presenting the specter of a global pandemic. Incidences of H5N1 outbreaks posed a host of questions concerning government capacity, transparency, and veracity in reporting.

The spread of COVID-19 across continents demonstrated how quickly outbreaks and pandemics can develop. It can be difficult to determine the severity, ease of transmission, and containment of a deadly virus. The unfamiliarity of the virus combined with its rapid spread makes coordination between the medical community, policymakers, and the media particularly important in combatting it. Organizations including the World Health Organization, the United Nations, and the Centers for Disease Control and Prevention and the National Institutes of Health in the US become involved during outbreaks. They monitor these outbreaks and provide information on symptoms and remedies. But is this enough? Experts also disagree on whether the media helps or hurts in educating the public about outbreaks, the role poverty plays in monitoring and containing pandemics, and the general effectiveness of surveillance and alert systems.

By studying previous pandemics and outbreaks, scientists have learned how to help guard against future outbreaks. But, as the world learned in 2020, these efforts are not always enough to help countries and communities be sufficiently prepared. As the viewpoints in *At Issue: COVID-19 and Other Pandemics* illustrate, the debate about the spread, prevention, and treatment of infectious deadly diseases is as contentious today as it was when the bubonic plague entered Constantinople.

Notes

1. Maria Cohut, Ph.D., "Global Impact of the COVID-19 Pandemic: 1 Year On," *Medical News Today*, March 12, 2021.
2. Martin Kettle, "A Century On, Why Are We Forgetting the Deaths of 100 Million?" *Guardian,* May 25, 2018.
3. Sarah Pruitt, "Microbe Behind Black Death Also Caused Devastating Plague 800 Years Earlier," History.com, August 30, 2018.
4. Kallie Szczepanski, "How the Black Death Started in Asia," ThoughtCo, August 12, 2019.
5. Tom James, "Black Death: The Lasting Impact," BBC, February 17, 2011.
6. Billy G. Smith, "The First Yellow Fever Pandemic: Slavery and Its Consequences," New York Academy of Medicine, October 15, 2018.
7. Joan Trossman Bien, "The Swine Flu Vaccine: 1976 Casts a Giant Shadow," Social Justice Foundation, June 14, 2017.
8. Joint United Nations Programme on HIV/AIDS, "The Global Strategy Framework on HIV/AIDS," 2001.
9. Ashish K. Jha, "The Ebola Outbreak: The Need for US Action," *Health Affairs,* October 2, 2019.
10. Arinjay Banerjee, "Explainer: What's the Difference Between an Outbreak and an Epidemic?" Conversation, January 7, 2015.

1

The COVID-19 Pandemic Required an Integrated National Response

Brian J. Gerber and Melanie Gall

Brian J. Gerber is associate professor at Watts College of Public Service and Community Solutions and co-director at the Center for Emergency Management and Homeland Security at Arizona State University. Melanie Gall is clinical professor and co-director at the Center for Emergency Management and Homeland Security at Arizona State University.

The United States was slow to respond to the COVID-19 outbreak in early 2020, despite warnings from abroad about the potential severity of the virus. Perhaps more consequential than a willingness to take the outbreak seriously was the Trump administration's response, which deviated from the emergency management practices that have been in place for national disasters for decades. By the end of the year, as the US death toll climbed and the economy staggered, the new Biden administration had changed the course of the country's strategy, returning to the established comprehensive federal disaster management practices.

"One Month In, How Biden Has Changed Disaster Management and the US COVID-19 Response," by Brian J. Gerber and Melanie Gall, The Conversation, February 18, 2021. https://theconversation.com/one-month-in-how-biden-has-changed-disaster -management-and-the-us-covid-19-response-155440. Licensed under CC BY-ND 4.0.

After one month in office, the Biden administration has fundamentally changed how the federal government responds to the COVID-19 pandemic.

In direct contrast to his predecessor, President Joe Biden is treating this as a national-scale crisis requiring a comprehensive national strategy and federal resources. If that sounds familiar, it should: It's a return to a traditional—and in many ways proven—approach to disaster management.

The Trump administration deviated dramatically from established emergency management practices. It politicized public health and related decision-making processes and overrode the disaster response roles of federal agencies, including the Centers for Disease Control and Prevention, the Department of Health and Human Services and the Federal Emergency Management Agency.

Among other things, the Trump administration established an entirely new coordination structure headed by a White House task force, then changed the lead federal agency from Health and Human Services to FEMA. Those moves, combined with a disjointed array of other operational task forces, made it difficult to create an integrated response. Even basic data collection from hospitals for tracking the coronavirus's spread was thrown into disarray by changes.

The Biden administration is now reempowering key federal agencies to return to the roles and responsibilities they were designed for within a planned national disaster management structure.

Our own work in hazards management, with both governments and nongovernmental organizations, has shown us that fidelity to proper process and respect for expertise is essential to effective disaster management. The Biden administration's approach to the pandemic so far suggests this is the model it will follow.

What Federal Emergency Response Was Designed to Do

By design, the US federal system for managing disasters is decentralized and tiered.

The system is structured so that local governments take the lead in managing hazards and responding to local emergencies. But when an emergency becomes a disaster-scale problem, state and federal governments should be prepared to provide financial assistance and other support, particularly logistical support.

FEMA, established in 1979 by President Jimmy Carter, has a crucial role as a national emergency management coordinator. Just getting all levels of government to work together effectively, along with private and nonprofit organizations, represents a massive challenge. Major crises over the years, including the Sept. 11 terror attacks, Hurricane Katrina in 2005 and Hurricane Sandy in 2012, have helped refine federal strategies and processes and improve preparedness for future disasters—including pandemics.

Pandemic preparedness has been a part of US emergency management planning since at least 2003. The H1N1 flu crisis in 2009 triggered the passage of the Pandemic and All-Hazards Preparedness Authorization Act in 2013. That law established Health and Human Services as the lead federal agency, and the statute specifically addresses the development of medical surge capacity, pandemic vaccine and drug development and more.

Managing a pandemic is more challenging than other types of disasters. Unlike a wildfire or tornado, which strikes a specific place for a limited period of time, a global pandemic is all-encompassing, affecting all jurisdictions and every economic sector. It requires focused coordination between public health and emergency response bureaucracies within government and with other key partners such as hospitals.

Given the scale of the COVID-19 pandemic, the federal government normally would have taken the lead in coordinating the response and assistance. Instead, the Trump administration devolved primary responsibility for the pandemic response to state and local governments, despite their limited capacity.

This approach was doomed to fail. It muddled use of the National Response Framework and created a competitive environment for state and local governments as they scrambled for supplies. It sidelined the agencies involved in pandemic preparedness, such as the CDC and the National Institute of Allergy and Infectious Diseases, and it ignored specific plans for a pandemic response. It also politicized resource allocation choices and undermined, through misinformation, the importance of public health behaviors such as wearing masks.

Biden's Return to Established Practices

Against this backdrop, the Biden administration's early efforts to return to established disaster management practice underscore the importance of leadership of complex systems used to address complex problems.

The list of changes in the month since Biden took office is extensive. The administration issued a comprehensive national strategy for pandemic response. It increased the involvement of FEMA and the Department of Defense to support vaccination distribution, expanded COVID-19 testing for underserved populations and rejoined the World Health Organization, which Trump had pulled out of. Biden also invoked the Defense Production Act to mobilize private industry to ramp up production of test kits, vaccines and personal protective equipment. The administration is now advocating for a national COVID-19 relief package in Congress.

The Biden administration's rapid, strategic reorientation of the federal government to manage the pandemic has parallels for other complex challenges, including developing a national strategy for addressing climate change. Continuing to refine these processes, including proper management of the federal bureaucracy, and public investments aimed at reducing risk should be priorities for the administration.

2

Defining Outbreaks, Epidemics, and Pandemics

Arinjay Banerjee

Arinjay Banerjee holds a PhD in virology and is a postdoctoral research fellow at McMaster University in Canada. He researches immune responses to viral infections along with health and public policy to address emerging infectious diseases.

Each infectious disease has a story to tell, but does it qualify as an epidemic? Is it an outbreak, or perhaps a pandemic? Defining each of these important terms allows one to frame an infectious disease and understand how its spread affects local communities, regions, and in some cases even multiple continents. These semantic differences also help to explain the nature of infectious diseases ranging from Ebola, which emerged as an outbreak and then advanced to an epidemic, to the COVID-19 virus, which also started out as an outbreak but advanced first to an epidemic and ultimately (and quickly) to a pandemic.

More than 8,000 people have died from Ebola in West Africa since February 2014 and it has spread beyond the three countries initially affected. So, it's an epidemic, right? Or is it an outbreak?

What about H1N1? The 2009 pandemic infected people around the world. But, so did the SARS epidemic in 2003. What's the difference between an epidemic and pandemic? What about diseases like malaria and Dengue? Dengue fever infects between 50 and 100 million people each year in countries all over the world. So that's the same thing as a pandemic? Not quite. Maybe you've seen headlines about West Nile Virus, Chikungunya fever or Middle East Respiratory Syndrome. And what are emerging and reemerging diseases?

It's time to brush up on the vocabulary that can help you understand just what infectious disease experts are trying to tell us.

Outbreaks, Epidemics, and Pandemics

An outbreak is the sudden occurrence of a disease in a community that has never experienced the disease before or when cases of that disease occur in numbers greater than expected in a defined area. The current Ebola scenario in West Africa started as an outbreak, which initially affected three countries.

So what exactly is an epidemic? It is an occurrence of a group of illnesses of similar nature and derived from a common source, in excess of what would be normally expected in a community or region. A classic example of an epidemic would be Severe Acute Respiratory Syndrome (SARS). The epidemic killed about 774 people out of 8,098 that were infected. It started as an outbreak in Asia and then spread to two dozen countries and took the form of an epidemic. The same is true for Ebola, which is now being termed an epidemic.

A pandemic on the other hand refers to a worldwide epidemic, which could have started off as outbreak, escalated to the level of an epidemic and eventually spread to a number of countries across continents. The 2009 flu pandemic is a good example. Between the period of April 2009 and August 2010, there were approximately 18,449 deaths in over 214 countries. The flu virus (H1N1) probably originated in Mexico, and within two months, sustained human-to-human transmission in several countries on different continents was reported, prompting the WHO to announce the highest alert level (phase 6, pandemic) on June 12, 2009.

Endemic Diseases

Some diseases can remain active in a given area for years and years. A disease is described as endemic when it is habitually present within a given geographic area. For example, Dengue, which is spread by mosquitoes, is endemic in more than 100 countries. So why isn't Dengue considered a pandemic yet? The point to consider here is that the Dengue cases are not from a common source. Mosquitoes do not fly beyond a few hundred meters, so the cases in each country are from a different source. Rotavirus-induced infant diarrhea is another example of an endemic disease, which is rampant in developing countries.

Emerging and Reemerging Diseases

We also come across words like "emerging" and "re-emerging." An emerging disease is one that has appeared in a population for the first time or one that may have existed before but is rapidly increasing in incidence. Examples of emerging infectious diseases are SARS, HIV and H1N1.

Despite advances made in the field of medicine, global travel has added to the complexity of controlling infectious diseases. Both the 2003 SARS epidemic and the 2009 H1N1 pandemic were spread to a large extent due to air travel.

Chikungunya is another viral disease that is emerging in the Western Hemisphere. The first known cases in the Western Hemisphere occurred around October 2013 among residents of the French side of St. Martin in the Caribbean. WHO confirmed more than 31,000 probable and confirmed cases, which were not imported but indigenous in nature, from numerous other Caribbean islands as of April 2014.

Middle East Respiratory Syndrome (MERS) emerged around April 2012 and has affected countries in the Middle East, Europe,

Africa, Asia and North America, with 945 human cases, including 348 deaths as of January 6, 2015.

Reemerging diseases are those that have historically infected humans but continue to appear in new locations or reappear after apparent control or elimination. Most of the reemerging disease agents appeared long ago and have survived and persisted in the environment. A classic example is the West Nile virus (WNV). It is thought that WNV arrived in the United States via an infected traveler, bird or mosquito, which entered America through air travel from the Middle East.

Why Bother?

Although people use terms like outbreak and epidemic interchangeably, it would only be fair to understand the definitive meaning behind each word. An outbreak can take the form of an epidemic and eventually a pandemic, but that does not entitle us to use these words incorrectly.

3

The Black Death of 1665 Devastated England, but It Started in China

Ben Johnson

Ben Johnson is an editor for History UK, *an online magazine about British history.*

The bubonic plague began its deadly path in China and spread to Europe. In England, diarist Samuel Pepys wrote about the disease and its effects on Londoners. It made its victims' skin turn black, which gave it the name "the Black Death." The name "bubonic" comes from the painful pockets of pus that formed on the body as a result of the disease. Folk remedies could not protect the many people succumbing to the disease, and the plague continued until cold weather hit. Could fleas have been the carrier and originator of this plague? This viewpoint examines that question and others.

In two successive years of the 17th century London suffered two terrible disasters. In the spring and summer of 1665 an outbreak of Bubonic Plague spread from parish to parish until thousands had died and the huge pits dug to receive the bodies were full. In 1666 the Great Fire of London destroyed much of the centre of London, but also helped to kill off some of the black rats and fleas that carried the plague bacillus.

Bubonic Plague was known as the Black Death and had been known in England for centuries. It was a ghastly disease.

"The Great Plague 1665—the Black Death," by Ben Johnson, Historic UK Ltd. Reprinted by permission.

The victim's skin turned black in patches and inflamed glands or "buboes" in the groin, combined with compulsive vomiting, swollen tongue and splitting headaches, made it a horrible, agonizing killer.

The plague started in the East, possibly China, and quickly spread through Europe. Whole communities were wiped out and corpses littered the streets as there was no one left to bury them.

It began in London in the poor, overcrowded parish of St. Giles-in-the-Field. It started slowly at first but by May of 1665, 43 had died. In June 6,137 people died, in July 17,036 people and at its peak in August, 31,159 people died. In all, 15% of the population perished during that terrible summer.

Incubation took a mere four to six days and when the plague appeared in a household, the house was sealed, thus condemning the whole family to death! These houses were distinguished by a painted red cross on the door and the words, "Lord have mercy on us." At night the corpses were brought out in answer to the cry, "Bring out your dead," put in a cart and taken away to the plague pits. One called the Great Pit was at Aldgate in London and another at Finsbury Fields.

The King, Charles II, and his Court left London and fled to Oxford. Those people who could sent their families away from London during these months, but the poor had no recourse but to stay.

In his diary, Samuel Pepys gives a vivid account of the empty streets in London, as all who could had left in an attempt to flee the pestilence.

It was believed that holding a posy of flowers to the nose kept away the plague and to this day judges are still given a nose-gay to carry on ceremonial occasions as a protection against the plague!

A song about the plague is still sung by children. "Ring-a-ring of roses" describes in great detail the symptoms of the plague and ends with "All fall down." The last word, "dead," is omitted today.

The plague spread to many parts of England. York was one city badly affected. The plague victims were buried outside the city walls and it is said that they have never been disturbed since then, as a precaution against a resurgence of the dreaded plague. The grassy embankments below the city walls are the sites of these plague pits.

A small village in Derbyshire called Eyam, 6 miles north of Bakewell, has a story of tragedy and courage that will always be remembered.

In 1665 a box of laundry was brought to Eyam by a traveller. The laundry was found to be infested with fleas, and the epidemic started.

80% of the people died here and there could have been a terrible outbreak in Derbyshire had the village not had a courageous rector called William Mompesson. He persuaded the villagers not to flee the village and so spread the infection, but to stay until the plague had run its course. His wife was one of the many victims and her tomb can be seen in Eyam churchyard.

Mompesson preached in the open air during the time of the plague, on a rock in a dell now called Cucklett Church. Every year a Commemorative Service is held here on the last Sunday in August. During their "siege" the villagers dropped money for provisions into a well so as not to spread the infection on the coins.

In some towns and villages in England there are still the old market crosses which have a depression at the foot of the stone cross. This was filled with vinegar during times of plague as it was believed that vinegar would kill any germs on the coins and so contain the disease.

The plague lasted in London until the late autumn when the colder weather helped kill off the fleas.

Over the centuries Bubonic Plague has broken out in Europe and the Far East. In 1900 there were outbreaks of plague in places as far apart as Portugal and Australia.

Influenza seems to be the modern form of plague. At the end of World War One an influenza outbreak circled the world during 1918–1919. Within a year 20 million people had died world-wide.

4

As Civilization Spread, So Did Smallpox

Centers for Disease Control and Prevention

The Centers for Disease Control and Prevention works to safeguard the United States from diseases, both foreign and domestic. It tracks and analyzes infectious diseases and shares information with the public.

Smallpox once was the scourge of civilization. Trade routes and colonization carried the disease around the world, and its victims suffered from fever, rashes, and death. Experiments with vaccination began in the late eighteenth century, and in the twentieth century, the World Health Organization (WHO) created a program to eliminate smallpox worldwide. The last cases occurred in the 1970s. WHO declared the world free of smallpox in 1980, which was considered to be among the greatest achievements in international public health.

The origin of smallpox is unknown. Smallpox is thought to date back to the Egyptian Empire around the 3rd century BCE (Before Common Era), based on a smallpox-like rash found on three mummies. The earliest written description of a disease that clearly resembles smallpox appeared in China in the 4th century CE (Common Era). Early written descriptions also appeared in India in the 7th century and in Asia Minor in the 10th century.

"History of Smallpox," Centers for Disease Control and Prevention.

Spread of Smallpox

The global spread of smallpox can be traced to the growth and spread of civilizations, exploration, and expanding trade routes over the centuries.

Historical Highlights

- 6th Century—Increased trade with China and Korea introduces smallpox into Japan.
- 7th Century—Arab expansion spreads smallpox into northern Africa, Spain, and Portugal.
- 11th Century—Crusades further spread smallpox in Europe.
- 15th Century—Portuguese occupation introduces smallpox into part of western Africa.
- 16th Century—European colonization and the African slave trade import smallpox into the Caribbean and Central and South America.
- 17th Century—European colonization imports smallpox into North America.
- 18th Century—Exploration by Great Britain introduces smallpox into Australia.

Early Control Efforts

Smallpox was a devastating disease. On average, 3 out of every 10 people who got it died. Those who survived were usually left with scars, which were sometimes severe.

One of the first methods for controlling the spread of smallpox was the use of variolation. Named after the virus that causes smallpox (variola virus), variolation is the process by which material from smallpox sores (pustules) was given to people who had never had smallpox. This was done either by scratching the material into the arm or inhaling it through the nose. With both types of variolation, people usually went on to develop the symptoms associated with smallpox, such as fever and a rash.

However, fewer people died from variolation than if they had acquired smallpox naturally.

The basis for vaccination began in 1796 when an English doctor named Edward Jenner observed that milkmaids who had gotten cowpox did not show any symptoms of smallpox after variolation. The first experiment to test this theory involved milkmaid Sarah Nelmes and James Phipps, the 9-year-old son of Jenner's gardener. Dr. Jenner took material from a cowpox sore on Nelmes' hand and inoculated it into Phipps' arm. Months later, Jenner exposed Phipps a number of times to variola virus, but Phipps never developed smallpox. More experiments followed, and, in 1801, Jenner published his treatise "On the Origin of the Vaccine Inoculation," in which he summarized his discoveries and expressed hope that "the annihilation of the smallpox, the most dreadful scourge of the human species, must be the final result of this practice."

Vaccination became widely accepted and gradually replaced the practice of variolation. At some point in the 1800s (the precise time remains unclear), the virus used to make the smallpox vaccine changed from cowpox to vaccinia virus.

Global Smallpox Eradication Program

In 1959, the World Health Organization (WHO) initiated a plan to rid the world of smallpox. Unfortunately, this global eradication campaign suffered from lack of funds, personnel, and commitment from countries, as well as a shortage of vaccine donations. Despite their best efforts, smallpox was still widespread in 1966, causing regular outbreaks in multiple countries across South America, Africa, and Asia.

The Intensified Eradication Program began in 1967 with a promise of renewed efforts. This time, laboratories in many countries where smallpox occurred regularly (endemic countries) were able to produce more, higher quality freeze-dried vaccine. A number of other factors also played an important role in the success of the intensified efforts, including the development of the bifurcated needle, establishment of a surveillance system to detect and investigate cases, and mass vaccination campaigns, to name a few.

By the time the Intensified Eradication Program began in 1967, smallpox had already been eliminated in North America (1952) and Europe (1953), leaving South America, Asia, and Africa (smallpox was never widespread in Australia). The Program made steady progress toward ridding the world of this disease, and by 1971 smallpox was eradicated from South America, followed by Asia (1975), and finally Africa (1977).

Last Cases of Smallpox

In late 1975, Rahima Banu, a three-year-old girl from Bangladesh, was the last person in the world to have naturally acquired variola major and the last person in Asia to have active smallpox. She was isolated at home with house guards posted 24 hours a day until she was no longer infectious. A house-to-house vaccination campaign within a 1.5 mile radius of her home began immediately, and every house, public meeting area, school, and healer within 5 miles was visited by a member of the Smallpox Eradication Program team to ensure the illness did not spread. A reward was also offered to anyone for reporting a smallpox case.

Ali Maow Maalin was the last person to have naturally acquired smallpox caused by variola minor. Maalin was a hospital cook in Merca, Somalia. On October 12, 1977, he accompanied two smallpox patients in a vehicle from the hospital to the local smallpox office. On October 22, he developed a fever. At first he was diagnosed with malaria, and then chickenpox. He was correctly diagnosed with smallpox by the smallpox eradication staff on October 30. Maalin was isolated and made a full recovery. Maalin died of malaria on July 22, 2013, while working in the polio eradication campaign.

Janet Parker was the last person to die of smallpox. It was 1978, and Parker was a medical photographer at the Birmingham University Medical School in England and worked one floor above the Medical Microbiology Department, where smallpox research was being conducted. She became ill on August 11 and developed a rash on August 15 but was not diagnosed with smallpox until 9 days later. She died on September 11, 1978. Her mother, who was providing care for her, developed smallpox on September 7, despite having been vaccinated on August 24. An investigation performed afterward suggested that Janet Parker had been infected either via an airborne route through the medical school building's duct system or by direct contact while visiting the microbiology corridor one floor above.

World Free of Smallpox

Almost two centuries after Jenner published his hope that vaccination could annihilate smallpox, on May 8, 1980, the 33rd World Health Assembly officially declared the world free of this disease. Eradication of smallpox is considered the biggest achievement in international public health.

Stocks of Variola Virus

Following the eradication of smallpox, scientists and public health officials determined there was still a need to perform research using the variola virus. They agreed to reduce the number of laboratories holding stocks of variola virus to only four locations. In 1981, the four countries that either served as a WHO collaborating center or were actively working with variola virus were the United States, England, Russia, and South Africa. By 1984, England and South Africa had either destroyed their stocks or transferred them to other approved labs. There are now only two locations where variola virus is officially stored and handled under WHO supervision: the Centers for Disease Control and Prevention in Atlanta, Georgia, and the State Research Center of Virology and Biotechnology (VECTOR Institute) in Koltsovo, Russia.

5

Flu Vaccines May Protect Only 60 Percent of People Who Receive It

Wayne C. Koff, Peter C. Doherty, and Margaret A. Hamburg

Wayne C. Koff is founder and CEO of the Human Vaccines Project in New York. Peter C. Doherty is an Australian immunologist who received the Nobel Prize in Physiology. Margaret A. Hamburg is the foreign secretary of the National Academy of Medicine in Washington, DC.

Despite the development of flu vaccines, the human immune system continues to render them ineffective. While it is true that vaccines have proven to be effective in eradicating smallpox, cholera, and other infectious diseases, the 2009 flu pandemic looked like it could have been a repeat of the 1918 flu pandemic that claimed some 50 million lives worldwide. Massive funding and years of research are the only effective means of decoding the human immune system and ridding the world of fatal infectious disease.

Last year was Australia's worst for flu since 2009. During the winter of 2017, which ended in August, there were 2.5 times more cases of influenza than in 2016, along with twice as many flu-related hospitalizations and twice as many flu-related deaths. This presaged the current influenza season in the Northern Hemisphere, which is on pace to be one of the worst in recent years. In addition,

"To Thwart Flu Pandemics, We Need to Decode the Human Immune System," by Wayne C. Koff, Peter C. Doherty, and Margaret A. Hamburg, Boston Globe Life Sciences Media, STAT, January 23, 2018. Reprinted by permission.

a simmering outbreak of an avian flu virus in China has killed 39 percent of nearly 1,600 persons infected since 2013. Those are two ominous signs as we mark the centennial of the greatest influenza outbreak in history, the 1918 flu pandemic that killed an estimated 50 million people around the world.

Public health experts have traditionally fought skirmishes against influenza. We believe that the time has come to mount an all-out assault on it by decoding the human immune system.

Every year, by tracking sentinel outbreaks throughout the world, public health officials try to stay one step ahead of influenza by developing a vaccine that will counter that season's strain. Yet even when the vaccine formulation hits the mark, it still confers protection in only about 60 percent of those who receive it. And it is often even less effective for those most at risk for influenza-related complications: young children, pregnant women, the elderly, and those with compromised immune systems.

History has repeatedly taught us that attempting to predict the next influenza pandemic, or chasing after potential pandemic outbreaks, can be both costly and ineffective. The primary reason that influenza vaccines aren't more effective, and the reason they can't generate broadly protective, long-lasting immunity in everyone, is that vaccines are thwarted by an entity we don't yet fully understand: the human immune system.

Make no mistake: Vaccines are among the most effective public health interventions in human history, second only to clean drinking water in the magnitude of their impact. They have led to the global eradication of one infectious disease, smallpox, and the near-eradication of polio. Vaccines have reduced death and disability caused by many infectious diseases, including measles, mumps, rubella, chickenpox, diphtheria, tetanus, and whooping cough. The vaccine against hepatitis B has reduced the incidence of liver cancer; those for human papillomavirus have done the same for cervical cancer.

But the full potential of vaccines remains just outside our reach. Some require multiple immunizations; others are less effective in the populations that need them the most, such as influenza vaccines in the elderly and diarrheal vaccines in the developing world. Vaccines against HIV, tuberculosis, and malaria still elude us, as these complex pathogens have developed mechanisms to evade the immune system that continue to impede vaccine developers. And we remain threatened by new and emerging infectious diseases such as Ebola and Zika, which will inevitably outpace the lengthy process of vaccine research and development, resulting in uncontrolled epidemics and leaving us woefully unprepared for the next global pandemic.

As recently as 2009, the world faced an influenza pandemic caused by what was, fortunately, a mild strain of influenza virus. By the time a vaccine was available specific to the strain, the flu had already spread to every continent, and was past its peak in North America. Had this strain of the influenza virus been severe, the outcome could have been catastrophic, mimicking the great pandemic of 1918.

Science is now poised to change all that. In the not-too-distant future, we predict that researchers will be able to harness the human immune system to prevent and control disease in ways previously considered unimaginable: one-shot vaccines that offer lifelong protection in everyone; a universal influenza vaccine that protects against seasonal and pandemic outbreaks of flu; vaccines against currently intractable infectious diseases; and, one day, vaccines against noninfectious chronic diseases, everything from cancer to heart disease and Alzheimer's disease.

Decoding the human immune system holds the key to the development of such new and improved vaccines. Deciphering the human immunome, the universal and common elements of the B and T cell receptors that make up the adaptive immune system, will facilitate germline targeting and structure-assisted vaccine discovery. Understanding the mechanisms for protective immunity will enable rational vaccine design aimed at specifically inducing such immune effector mechanisms.

This is finally possible because of the convergence of technological advances across biomedical, computer, and engineering sciences, including the enhancement of artificial intelligence and machine learning capabilities to analyze and interpret unprecedented quantities of data. In the same way that the Human Genome Project transformed biomedical research and enabled the genesis of personalized medicine, and the Hubble Telescope transformed planetary sciences and our understanding of the universe, decoding the human immune system has the potential to revolutionize 21st century global health, ushering in new advances in diagnostics, vaccines and therapeutics.

It won't be cheap, and it won't be easy. Decoding the human immune system will take a decade of research and cost more than $1 billion. It will require innovative public-private partnerships working collectively to decipher the common components and rules of human immunity. But the return on investment—a blueprint for how the immune system fights disease—will be extraordinary and applicable to all facets of human health.

Deciphering how the human immune system combats disease is one of the greatest frontiers of science, and is now within reach. If society grasps this unprecedented opportunity, commits resources to it, and facilitates creative new models for working together across multiple scientific disciplines, we can not only eliminate the threat of pandemic influenza but reshape how we approach all life-threatening diseases.

6

The COVID-19 Pandemic Was Politicized at the Expense of Science

Laura K. Field

Laura K. Field is a writer and political theorist and scholar in residence at American University. Her academic writing spans antiquity and modernity and has appeared in the Journal of Politics, *the* Review of Politics, *and* Polity.

The year 2020 saw an extraordinary convergence of science, politics, and social justice. The COVID-19 pandemic ravaged the United States and much of the world, and while many people looked to science for answers, then president Donald Trump promoted antiscience and misinformation in order to boost his own standing. At the same time, Black Lives Matter protests swept America, reflecting a severely divided nation. The dangerous combination of a deadly pandemic, an authoritarian president, and calls for police reform created a troubling environment that was eventually somewhat mitigated by the election of President Joe Biden.

It has been a disorienting few weeks for anyone interested in the relationship between knowledge and power. For months now, since the start of the pandemic, Americans have experienced the brutal consequences of an administration deeply distrustful of expertise. As we tracked the virus' spread, and watched the death toll mount—especially in our most vulnerable communities and at-risk populations—many wondered: why are some of the most powerful people in the country so indifferent to science, and by extension, to human life?

At the end of May, Americans witnessed a still more vivid horror in the video of George Floyd's killing at the hand of four Minneapolis police officers. In subsequent weeks, our streets were rightly filled with protests, as well as riots and more police violence. Of course, the reversal concerning public life was jarring, and led to more bewilderment. What about the pandemic? What happened to science's authority? Does any of that matter anymore? With Trump set to start-in on campaign rallies again, the questions linger.

There are serious discussions to be had here—about racism and police brutality, the politicization of knowledge, the civic imperatives of scientists and experts, and how good political decisions are made. But before conceding too much to charges of liberal hypocrisy and the destruction of scientific credibility in the wake of the George Floyd protests—charges that are widespread on the right, and have taken shape across the media landscape since the protests began—it's worth recollecting the broader context. After all, the Trump-supporting right has a distinctive set of ideas regarding the proper relationship between expertise and power. Sophisticated thinkers in Trump's orbit made these plain throughout the coronavirus crisis.

When it comes to the pandemic, elite intellectuals on the right leveraged two particular insights to lend cover and legitimacy to the president. The first has to do with the uncertain nature of science, and the second is about the exceptional character of political action and statecraft. Taken together, these insights amount to the highbrow version of Trump's perennial claims to political genius. But whether it's Trump, or Laura Ingraham, or Peter Navarro, or Richard Epstein, the basic thought is always the same: I may not be a doctor or epidemiologist, but the science is uncertain, and I've got that certain je-ne-sais-quoi that gives me a superior understanding.

Unlike with full-on conspiracy theories, these clever arguments work, when they do, because they contain real kernels of truth. Science does need to be interpreted by political actors, after all, and some people have better political judgment than others. But a closer look at the most sophisticated versions of these claims can help us to see how little truths are sometimes put in the service of much bigger lies. This is a set of ideas that denigrates expertise and professes respect for dynamic political action, but which ends up empowering ignorance and denigrating civic virtue. As we form our judgements about ongoing events, we need to keep this stark reality in mind.

Truth and Uncertainty

Statements showcasing the uncertain character of knowledge often serve to discredit science and expertise, but they echo a skepticism that real experts share. The scientific endeavor is, for all of its successes and achievements, complicated, multifaceted, and often quite fraught. It is the nature of modern inquiry to push forward into uncertain terrain, and it is always subject to critique and revision. Late in the 19th Century, Max Weber put it this way, "Every scientific 'fulfilment' raises new 'questions'; it asks to be 'surpassed' and outdated."

Furthermore, scientific disciplines operate on different dimensions of a given question, so experts often talk past one another. As Professor Sheila Jasanoff explains in a recent interview about the pandemic: "Someone who understands the dynamics of what happens inside a family when you're cooped up together for week upon week—that person is not going to tell you very much about how a virus acts inside a body, or how quickly contagion spreads if you don't self-isolate." Back in 2000, Daniel Sarewitz speaks of a similar phenomenon, the "excess of objectivity," arguing that "science is sufficiently rich, diverse, and Balkanized to provide comfort and support for a range of subjective, political positions on complex issues." At bottom, science is always a human activity. Scientific evidence can be used in the service of false ideas, like biological racism, and, of course, some scientists are just plain corrupt.

Throughout the pandemic, the Covid-questioners exploited the all-too-human character of science to undercut the authority of epidemiologists and policy-makers (as others have observed, there is much here that resembles the climate-denier playbook). From the pages of the *American Mind*, we heard about the "hazy scientific evidence" surrounding mask-wearing, and learned that expert analysis "is often in dispute and uncertain," to the point that "all 'sides' arguing right now use models and numbers as they wish." In *First Things*, we heard about how "expertise provides no immunity against the desire for power," and that the "politics of science" is "no more innocent than regular politics." At the height of the anti-lockdown protests, Sohrab Ahmari wrote about how "They Blinded Us With Science." According to his "History of a Delusion," most people in our "post-Enlightenment" culture believe that science explains everything, and it has taken Covid-19 to show them otherwise. "There is nothing quite like a sudden and unforeseen pandemic to puncture the confidence of confident men," he writes with satisfaction.

None of this will surprise anyone who follows elite conservative thinking, where disdain for mainstream experts (or "liberalocrats," or the "technocratic elite," or "urban-gentry liberals") is something of a sacramental duty. But in each case we can see a distortion. It's true, I think, that scientism (the belief that science will solve everything) is blinkered, but that doesn't make everyone a "post-Enlightenment" ideologue. Few indeed are immune to power's allure, but that doesn't make everyone equally likely to pursue it. And it's true that science involves uncertainty, and epidemiological modeling notoriously so, but that does not preclude the possibility of arriving at meaningful agreement and consensus.

Compared with most social and political phenomena (the climate crisis, say, or racism, police brutality, and widespread civic unrest), the pandemic is relatively concrete and tangible. Daniel Sarewitz is hardly one to flatter the scientific community, but even he put it like this, back in March: "COVID-19 is a hard problem, but not a complex one. We know what COVID-19 is because we see it around us." This does not make dealing with a pandemic simple. It does mean that experts understood, at the outset of the crisis and along the way, which concrete actions could have alleviated the devastation caused by the virus.

Trump's intellectual defenders on the right waved away this knowledge and minimized these options, further eroding public trust in science and good government.

From Denial to Political Triumphalism

With the climate crisis, science talk on the right begins and ends with denialism; with Covid-19, though, it's more like a throat-clearing exercise. Once the scientists, technocrats, and policy wonks have been dismissed, the real heroes are welcomed onstage—the hypothetical Statesmen, Rulers, and Mensch who will lead us into greatness. Overall, the message among intellectual elites on the right tends to be quite hopeful: we need not attend to elite experts because there's something out there that's way better. Science is dreadfully uncertain, but politics doesn't have to be.

Pierre Manent gives us a textbook example of this mode of thinking in an alarmist interview that appeared in *First Things* at the end of April. Manent is sometimes thoughtful about liberalism and modernity, and was very critical of the European lockdowns. When the interviewer leadingly suggests that politics should stand "on its own," so as to "triumph" above expertise, Manent takes the opportunity to expound upon what real leadership—in contradistinction to the European reality—would look like: "It is up to elected officials to make decisions because they are the ones who are in charge of the whole, that is, the body politic; it is up to them to take all parameters into account and to envision all the consequences of their actions. Aristotle was right: Politics is the queen of the sciences!" Having denigrated the actual politicians in charge, during a deadly pandemic, Manent appeals to this higher, classical notion of politics as an alternative. The prudent

Aristotelian would have acted differently, enjoying a more synoptic view; they would not have deferred to the technocrats.

I do not begrudge Manent his concerns about civil liberties. What is more, I find Aristotle's insights into political action highly appealing. Aristotle suggests that political knowledge is the most authoritative (or "architectonic") kind of knowledge because it has the biggest scope, and can do the most good for human beings. It's a high-minded and dynamic depiction of political agency—one that makes a clear case for the power of synoptic understanding, and likely to speak to anyone frustrated by bureaucracies, gridlock, and wonks. It's always worth reminding ourselves that political actors have to make challenging, impactful decisions in a way that scientists and technocrats typically do not. Aristotle teaches that good political thinking is flexible: decisions and judgments must be made with partial knowledge, as circumstances change.

But none of it is an excuse to scrap the science. There is a universe of difference between "I hear and appreciate all of these insights, and will make my decision keeping all of these important considerations in mind" and "This information is complicated and uncertain, so I'm just going to go with my gut." There's a world of difference between thoughtful incorporation of trusted information, and the hasty rejection of it. And there's a vast chasm separating fair-minded political critique from sophistry that gives cover to idiocy.

I don't think Manent falls into the latter category. However, it's hard to reconcile how a thoughtful person wouldn't understand why dramatic—if imperfect—action was a necessary response to the Covid crisis. When it comes to Trump's defenders here at home, however, it's hard to be charitable. Like Manent, the most sophisticated among them have been eager to discuss the proper role of the statesman in times of pandemic. They all seem to agree that science and technocratic expertise don't contribute much to that role.

Among the clearest examples of this anti-intellectual view of statesmanship come from The Claremont Institute (the group that published Michael Anton's "The Flight 93 Election," and has been giving intellectual succour to Trump ever since). Writing in the institute's flagship publication, the *Claremont Review of Books*, Professor Charles R. Kesler has spoken of Trump in terms befitting a high-level statesman, and speaks positively of the president's dislike for "the airs and claims of experts, detached from and above the subjects of their experiments." Early in the pandemic, Matthew Peterson—the institute's VP for education—showed high hopes for Trump's pandemic leadership precisely because the president is unbound by "calcified ideological frameworks" and willing to flout conventional expertise. Writing in *American Mind*—the institute's lesser publication, Peterson declares that this is "A Time for Statesmanship." He bemoans America's lack of statesmanship in terms that recall Manent's anti-technocratic gambit ("We don't believe in statesmanship anymore, really. We don't know what that is. But 'data-driven decision making' can't substitute for it, or evade politics in the broadest sense"). Then, with a gesture to Machiavelli ("leaders harness fortuna"), he describes his ideal type of political man. We need someone with the "competence, courage, and vision to lead us decisively to victory." Only Trump, Peterson concludes, can "bring us into a new century of greatness"—and eventually he will, we learn, "because he must."

(Last week the noble leaders of The Claremont Institute took it upon themselves to pronounce that "America is Not Racist." That is just a lie peddled by elites who are determined to destroy the country.)

And the gentlemen at Claremont aren't alone in their high hopes for Trump's performance during the pandemic. Victor Davis Hanson was enthusiastic about the president's potential in the crisis—again, precisely because of his skepticism of expertise. In March Hanson remarked that the president ought to model himself on the ancients, and make a display of his "terrific strategic foresight" to defeat the coronavirus. Hanson said: "Trump must have the right information but also the instincts to determine which expert advice is suspect and which is inspired, and which orthodox recommendation is wrong and which unorthodox alternative is right." In a more serious article for *First Things*, Nathan Pinkoski writes about what true political decision-making should entail. Pinkoski worries that "managerial experts" lack "an adequate understanding of the hierarchy of human goods." He counsels deference to those "non-managerial, non-expert leaders" who hold political office, and therefore provide "a more integrated account of the good, one that is based on wisdom, not expertise." We should trust the political leaders, not the experts, since they are the ones with real values and wisdom.

There is a lot to say here—about policy-making, the appropriate role of contentious views, different kinds of political virtue, and wishful thinking. Suffice it to say that Trump's Covid-19 response did not live up to these vaunted expectations.

From Triumphalism to Fatalism

It is not hard to imagine what responsible, energetic American leadership through the Covid-19 crisis would have looked like. It would have begun with a leader who had listened to epidemiologists' warnings and started to prepare the country for a potential health crisis back in January. A responsible person would have been upfront about the problems that lockdowns pose for civil liberties in free societies. She would have moved early to protect vulnerable populations, as well as the 2020 elections. A good, respectable leader would understand that politics, the economy, and the pandemic are intertwined, and so would have sought ways to reopen that maximally protect people's health and freedoms. Trump's elite entourage is right that this would have required her to have great foresight, courage, and energy, and I'll be the first to admit that it's unfair to hold our president up to such a fantastical imaginary ideal. But it's helpful to know, in a concrete way, that things might have gone quite differently, and how.

In the end, Trump's elite enablers understood that he isn't a perfect vessel, and so they dodged and hedged their bets. They did this by staying quiet, or by returning to the theme of uncertainty and indeterminacy—not only in science, but also now in political and metaphysical affairs. Peterson made sure to note that "Big decisions are hard because they are risky—and their outcomes will be messy regardless of what is decided." Princeton historian Allen C. Guelzo suggested that it was unreasonable to expect Trump to have much of a role in the pandemic at all, since some of his predecessors didn't exert themselves about such things. For a while, Professor Hanson was convinced that America's approach to the pandemic was working. One month later, though, he was blaming America's high-level experts for all kinds of confusion, and soon was putting the onus for recovery squarely on the public: "Americans must master their fears of the virus and dare to go back to work." In this, he echoed the brutal fatalism of R. R. Reno, who warned early on against an "ill-conceived crusade against human finitude and the dolorous reality of death." So much for political virtue or statesmanship. Que sera sera.

Today, we face 115,000 dead souls—a number that, if more Americans had listened to the president's instincts instead of their own good sense, could have been far higher, and which continues to rise. As any sensible person must acknowledge, we are likely to see new spikes in cases as a result of the massive protests that have roiled the country. But that doesn't mean that liberals and leftists have suddenly rejected science and expertise. For one thing, the civil protests have launched an agonized but good-faith discussion among scientists and in the media about the interplay of scientific expertise, human values, and political action. This is an entirely necessary conversation that parallels ongoing debates throughout civil society about the moral valence of modern (typically "neutral") professional life.

More importantly, the protests themselves—massive, mostly peaceful protests, in every state, and around the world—have been a global exercise in the kind of dynamic, political reasoning that the intellectual right is constantly professing to admire. While there has been destruction and violence—by rioters as well as the police—mostly we have seen a powerful expression of political solidarity and a moving call to justice. Meanwhile, today's right is so entranced by their caricature of coddled, data-obsessed liberals that they could not see the protesters for what they are: not a bunch of flip-flopping technocrats, but civic-minded people taking discernable risks in the fight for a better, antiracist future. Similarly, the right's views on political authority are so fusty, authoritarian, and delusional, that they can hardly conceive of free-thinking people making real political judgments of their own.

This is a worldview in which experts are reviled and authoritarians coddled, a way of thinking that regularly pits raw force against truth, against knowledge, and against our equal freedoms. It's a universe where lying projections of MAGA greatness and real state-sanctioned violence are prized more highly than the informed actions of a free-thinking citizenry.

It's closed off from what is best in politics. Don't fall for it now.

7

Medical Professionals Must Unite Against Anti-Vaccination Movement

Azhar Hussain, Syed Ali, Madiha Ahmed, and Sheharyar Hussain

Azhar Hussain is associated with the College of Health Professionals at Davenport University in Grand Rapids, Michigan. Syed Ali is affiliated with the Department of Psychology at Stony Brook University in Stony Brook, New York. Madiha Ahmed is associated with the Department of Medicine at Touro College of Osteopathic Medicine in New York, New York. Sheharyar Hussain is with the Department of Clinical Psychology at Teachers College, Columbia University in New York, New York.

Campaigns to promote the anti-vaccine movement have led to decreases in the number of vaccinations and outbreaks of infectious diseases—such as measles—previously believed to have been eliminated. With the widespread availability of information online, especially through social media, patients claim to share authority with their physicians and make their own possibly deadly decisions about whether to vaccinate those at risk of disease, including young children. (Similar conflicts arose as the COVID-19 vaccines were rolled out.) Medical professionals, researchers, governments, and educators must unite in their efforts to fight against anti-vaccination movements and their misinformation.

"The Anti-Vaccination Movement: A Regression in Modern Medicine," by Azhar Hussain, Syed Ali, Madiha Ahmed, and Sheharyar Hussain, Cureus, July 1, 2018. https://www .cureus.com/articles/13250-the-anti-vaccination-movement-a-regression-in-modern -medicine. Licensed under CC BY 4.0.

V accines are one of the most important measures of preventative medicine to protect the population from diseases and infections. They have contributed to decreasing rates of common childhood diseases and, in some cases, have even wiped out some diseases that were common in years past, such as smallpox, rinderpest, and have nearly eradicated polio.[1] In fact, according to the World Health Organization's Polio Global Eradication Initiative, the inactivated polio vaccine (IPV) will be used as a backbone for eradicating poliovirus in the next decade. However, there has been a recent rise in anti-vaccination sentiments surrounding beliefs that vaccines cause more harm than benefits to the health of the children who receive them. The premise of the anti-vaccination movement can also be contributed to the demonization of vaccinations by news and entertainment outlets. Voices such as Jenny McCarthy's have proven to be influential, sweeping fear and distrust into parents' minds by parading as "autism experts." Social media and television talk show hosts, such as Oprah Winfrey, played a big role in this miseducation by giving credence to the campaign. This has caused vaccination rates to sustain a surprising drop in some Western countries.[2] The decrease in vaccinations has led to recent outbreaks of diseases that were thought to be "eliminated," such as measles. Still, other reasons for the anti-vaccination movement can be due to personal reasons, such as religious or secular views. A drop in immunizations poses a threat to the herd immunity the medical world has worked hard to achieve. Global communities are now more connected than ever, which translates to a higher probability of the transmission of pathogens. The only thing that can protect populations against a rapidly spreading disease is the disease's resistance created by herd immunity when the majority are immune after vaccinations. Given the highly contagious nature of diseases like measles, vaccination rates of 96% to 99% are necessary to preserve herd immunity and prevent future outbreaks.[3]

Origins of the Anti-Vaccination Movement

Fear of vaccines and myths against them are not a new phenomenon. Opposition to vaccines goes as far back as the 18th century when, for example, Reverend Edmund Massey in England called the vaccines "diabolical operations" in his 1772 sermon, "The Dangerous and Sinful Practice of Inoculation."[4] He decried these vaccines as an attempt to oppose God's punishments upon man for his sins.[5] Similar religious opposition was seen in the "New World" even earlier, such as in the writings of Reverend John Williams in Massachusetts, who also cited similar reasons for his opposition to vaccines claiming that they were the devil's work.[6] However, opposition against vaccines was not only manifested in theological arguments; many also objected to them for political and legal reasons. After the passage of laws in Britain in the mid-19th century making it mandatory for parents to vaccinate their children, anti-vaccine activists formed the Anti-Vaccination League in London. The league emphasized that its mission was to protect the liberties of the people, which were being "invaded" by Parliament and its compulsory vaccination laws.[7] Eventually, the pressure exerted by the league and its supporters compelled the British Parliament to pass an act in 1898, which removed penalties for not abiding by vaccination laws and allowed parents who did not believe vaccination was beneficial or safe to not have their children vaccinated.[8] Since the rise and spread of the use of vaccines, opposition to vaccines has never completely gone away, vocalized intermittently in different parts of the world due to arguments based in theology, skepticism, and legal obstacles.[9]

Anti-Vaccination Propaganda

While pushback against the measles vaccine due to fears of its connection to autism is the most recent example that comes to mind, there have been other instances of outbreaks of previously "extinct" diseases in modern times. One example is the refusal of some British parents to vaccinate their children in the 1970s and 1980s against pertussis in response to the publication of a report in 1974 that credited 36 negative neurological reactions to the whole-cell pertussis vaccine.[10] This caused a decrease in the pertussis vaccine uptake in the United Kingdom (UK) from 81% in 1974 to 31% in 1980, eventually resulting in a pertussis outbreak in the UK, putting severe strain and pressure on the National Health System.[11, 12] Vaccine uptake levels were elevated to normal levels after the publication of a national reassessment of vaccine efficacy that reaffirmed the vaccine's benefits, as well as financial incentives for general practitioners who achieved the target of vaccine coverage.[13] Disease incidence declined dramatically as a result.

The anti-vaccination movement was most strongly rejuvenated in recent years by the publication of a paper in the *Lancet* by a former British doctor and researcher, Andrew Wakefield, which suggested credence to the debunked-claim of a connection between the measles, mumps, and rubella (MMR) vaccine and development of autism in young children.[14] Several studies published later disproved a causal association between the MMR vaccine and autism.[15–18] Wakefield drew severe criticism for his flawed and unethical research methods, which he used to draw his data and conclusions.[19] A journalistic investigation also revealed that there was a conflict of interest with regard to Wakefield's publication because he had received funding from litigants against vaccine manufacturers, which he obviously did not disclose to either his co-workers nor medical authorities.[20] For all of the aforementioned reasons, the *Lancet* retracted the study, and its editor declared it "utterly false."[21] As a result, three months later, he was also struck off the UK Medical Registry, barring him from practicing medicine in the UK. The verdict declared that he had "abused his position of trust" and "brought the medical profession into disrepute" in the studies he carried out.[22]

Repercussions of Declining Vaccination Rates

The damage, however, was already done and the myth was spread to many different parts of the world, especially Western Europe and North America. In the UK, for example, the MMR vaccination rate dropped from 92% in 1996 to 84% in 2002. In 2003, the rate was as low as 61% in some parts of London, far below the rate needed to avoid an epidemic of measles.[23] In Ireland, in 1999–2000, the national immunization level had fallen below 80%, and in part of North Dublin, the level was around 60%.[24] In the US, the controversy following the publication of the study led to a decline of about 2% in terms of parents obtaining the MMR vaccine for their children in 1999 and 2000. Even after later studies explicitly and thoroughly debunked the alleged MMR-autism link, the drop in vaccination rates persisted.[25]

As a result, multiple breakouts of measles have occurred throughout different parts of the Western world, infecting dozens of patients and even causing deaths. In the UK in 1998, 56 people contracted measles; in 2006, this number increased to 449 in the first five months of the year, with the first death since 1992.[26] In 2008, measles was declared endemic in the UK for the first time in 14 years.[27] In Ireland, an outbreak occurred in 2000 and 1,500 cases and three deaths were reported. The outbreak was reported to have occurred as a direct result of a drop in vaccination rates following the MMR controversy.[28] In France, more than 22,000 cases of measles were reported from 2008–2011.[29] The United States has not been an exception, with outbreaks occurring most recently in 2008, 2011, and 2013.[30–32]

Perhaps the most infamous example of a measles outbreak in the United States occurred in 2014–2015. The outbreak was believed to originate from the Disneyland Resort in Anaheim, California, and resulted in an estimated 125 people contracting the disease.[33] It was estimated that MMR vaccination rates among the exposed population in which secondary cases have occurred might be as low as 50% and likely no higher than 86%.[34] Physicians in the region were criticized for deviating from the CDC's (Centers for Disease Control and Prevention) recommended vaccination schedule and/or discouraging vaccination. As a result, California passed Senate Bill 277, a mandatory vaccination law in June 2015, banning personal and religious exemptions to abstain from vaccinations.[35]

Technology and Its Effects on Anti-Vaccination Movement

Access to medical information online has dramatically changed the dynamics of the healthcare industry and patient-physician interactions. Medical knowledge that was previously bound to textbooks and journals, or held primarily by medical professionals, is now accessible to the layman, which has shifted the power from doctors as exclusive managers of a patient's care to the patients themselves.[36] This has led to the recent establishment of shared decision-making between patients and healthcare physicians.[37] While this is beneficial in some ways, the dissemination of false and misleading information found on the internet can also lead to negative consequences, such as parents not giving consent to having their children vaccinated. When it comes to vaccines, the false information is plentiful and easy to find. An analysis of YouTube videos about immunization found that 32% opposed vaccination and that these had higher ratings and more views than pro-vaccine videos.[38] An analysis of MySpace blogs about HPV immunization found that 43% portrayed the immunization in a negative light; these blogs referenced vaccine-critical organizations and cited inaccurate data.[39] A similar study of Canadian internet users tracked the sharing of influenza vaccine information on social media networks, such as Facebook, Twitter, YouTube, and Digg. Of the top search results during the study period, 60% promoted anti-vaccination sentiments.[40] A study that examined the content of the first 100 anti-vaccination sites found after searching for "vaccination" and "immunization" on Google concluded that 43% of websites were anti-vaccination (including all of the first 10).[41]

Online anti-vaccination authors use numerous tactics to further their agendas. These tactics include, but are not limited to, skewing science, shifting hypotheses, censoring opposition, attacking critics, claiming to be "pro-safe vaccines," and not "anti-vaccine," claiming that vaccines are toxic or unnatural, and more.[42] Not only are these tactics deceitful and dishonest, they are also effective on many parents. A study that evaluated how effectively users assessed the accuracy of medical information about vaccines online concluded that 59% of student participants thought retrieved sites were entirely accurate; however, out of the 40 sites they were given, only 18 were actually accurate, while 22 were inaccurate. These sites were not evidence-based and argued vaccines were inherently dangerous without any merit-based argument. More than half of participants (53%) left the exercise with significant misconceptions about vaccines.[43] Research has also shown that viewing an anti-vaccine website for merely 5–10 minutes increased perceptions of vaccination risks and decreased perceptions of the risks of vaccine omission, compared to visiting a control site.[44] The study also found that the anti-vaccine sentiments obtained from viewing the websites still persisted five months later, causing the children of these parents to obtain fewer vaccinations than recommended.[45] The role of the online access to false anti-vaccination information just cannot be understated in examining the rise and spread of the anti-vaccination movement.

Ethical and Legal Issues Regarding Vaccination

Opposition to the MMR vaccine among parents leads to an ethical dilemma that can be analyzed using both medical ethics and moral principles. Medical ethics call for health professionals to abide by a code of bioethics upholding autonomy, non-maleficence, beneficence, and justice. The most relevant in mandating vaccinations are autonomy and non-maleficence.[46] Patients are entitled to the right to refuse vaccination using "our children, our choice" based on their autonomy, while health care providers are morally obligated to treat everyone with non-maleficence and avoiding harm to society at all costs.

At the individual level, religion is a common reason to refuse vaccination. The MMR vaccine specifically has been the cause of instigating debate among the Hindu, Protestant, Orthodox Jewish, and Jehovah's Witness communities. Specific religious views on vaccines in general, however, are not normally the cause for debate but instead the components of the MMR vaccine.[47] The MMR vaccine, combined with the rubella vaccine, was originally derived from the cells of aborted fetal tissue. Hindu, Protestant, Muslim, and Jewish communities are generally opposed to abortion for moral reasons based on religious teachings; thus, individuals from these beliefs may cite religious reasons for filing vaccine exemptions. Further, the MMR vaccine contains porcine gelatin as a stabilizer, a means for ensuring effective storage. The porcine ingredients are unlike gelatins used for oral consumption and purified down to small peptides, commonly used in medicine capsules as well.[48] As there is a wide range of practice preferences in every religion, some individuals belonging to religions, such as Judaism, Islam, and Hinduism (to name a few), may be opposed to injecting a porcine product into their body along with the vaccine.[47] Further, other religious views, such as the ones held by Dutch-Protestant Christian congregations, consider vaccinations "inappropriate meddling in the work of God." These groups, therefore, believe that we should not change the predestined fate of someone who becomes ill.[49]

While exercising autonomy and refusing vaccination is valid for sensitive personal issues, it will cause more harm than good if a certain percentage of the population does not get vaccines causing the immunization rate to fall below the herd immunity threshold. This threshold varies in every disease. The development of vaccines is considered one of the greatest strides made in medicine due to the enormous benefits to an entire population. From an ethics perspective, achieving herd immunity and minimizing the amount of "freeloaders" is in the best interest of society as a whole.[48, 49]

Further, studies liken the decision to object to vaccinations to military service drafts. For the conscientious objectors, military duty and receiving a vaccine hold the same costs: liberty, personal risk, and utility in terms of time.[41] Naturally, the costs of military duty are more taxing and demand more from an individual than receiving a vaccine. In terms of herd immunity and depending on the severity of impending diseases, these costs are ones that they should incur for the benefit of themselves as well as society.

At the forefront of the legal complications lies the state-regulated vaccinations for all children attending school. Anti-vaccination proponents argue that this is an infringement upon autonomy; however, public health policymakers justify their actions using rule utilitarianism. Rule utilitarianism is the ideology that a rule for society should be established that has the best outcome for the greatest amount of people in the society. In addition to this, John Stuart Mill's essay "On Liberty" explains the Harm Principle that is often used to justify mandated infectious disease control methods, including vaccines.[50] The Harm Principle justifies interfering with autonomy and individual liberties, against their will, if it is done so as to prevent harm to others. An example of this was seen in California in 2014–2015 after an outbreak of measles led to the passing of Senate Bill 277 calling for state-mandated vaccinations for everyone—no personal exemptions. The root of the problem, however, was most likely to be contributed to Wakefield's fraudulent findings striking the fear of a vaccination-autism link in parents, which led to an all-time low rate of people receiving the MMR vaccine. The hoax has been called the most damaging medical hoax in 100 years after bringing about outbreaks of diseases otherwise eradicated.[8, 9, 11]

In the times that we have achieved herd immunity, there remain two questions then. Can legal exemptions still be justified? And should these exemptions be limited to religious reasons or should they include secular reasoning as well?[21, 25] Most scientists and medical experts suggest that exemptions should only even be considered if society is well within the limits for herd immunity.

As for the religious versus secular debate, it is difficult to ignore secular objections as most of them are rooted in spiritual or holistic personal views.[6, 47] Since herd immunity is cumulative, the ability to waive immunizations is concluded to be difficult but not impossible. If the waivers are given to a small number of individuals who sincerely need them rather than ones who are inconvenienced by them, waivers may be ethically and legally sound.

Conclusions

The rise of anti-vaccination movements in parts of the Western world poses a dire threat to people's health and the collective herd immunity. People of all ages have fallen victim to recent outbreaks of measles, one of the most notable "eliminated" diseases that made a comeback as a direct consequence of not reaching the immunization threshold for MMR vaccines. These outbreaks not only put a strain on national healthcare systems but also cause fatal casualties. Therefore, it is of the utmost importance that all stakeholders in the medical world—physicians, researchers, educators, and governments—unite to curb the influence of the anti-vaccination movement targeting parents. Research has shown that even parents favorable to vaccination can be confused by the ongoing debate, leading them to question their choices. Many parents lack basic knowledge of how vaccines work, as well as access to accurate information explaining the importance of the process. Furthermore, those with the greatest need for knowledge about vaccination seem most vulnerable to this information. Further, we must effectively combat the wrongful demonization of vaccinations through social media and news media platforms. A qualitative study that explored how parents respond to competing media messages about vaccine safety concluded that personal experiences, value systems, and level of trust in health professionals are essential to parental decision making about immunization. Therefore, to combat the anti-vaccination movement, there must be a strong emphasis on helping parents develop trust in health professionals and relevant authorities, educating them on the facts and figures, debunking the myths peddled by the anti-vaccination movements, and even introducing legislation that promotes vaccination, if not mandating it.

References

1. Achievements in Public Health, 1900–1999 Impact of Vaccines Universally Recommended for Children—United States, 1990–1998. (1999). Accessed: June 17, 2018: http://www.cdc.gov/mmwr/preview/mmwrhtml/00056803.htm.
2. Anderson P: Another media scare about MMR vaccine hits Britain. *BMJ.* 1999, 318:1578. 10.1136/bmj.318.7198.1578
3. Plans-Rubió P: Evaluation of the establishment of herd immunity in the population by means of serological surveys and vaccination coverage. *Hum Vaccin Immunother.* 2012, 8:184-88. 10.4161/hv.18444
4. Massey E: Sermon against the dangerous and sinful practice of inoculation. Preach'd at St. Andrew's Holborn, on Sunday, July the 8th, 1722. / By Edmund Massey, M.A. Lecturer of St. Alban Woodstreet. Gale Ecco, Print Editions. 2010, Accessed: June 17, 2018: http://name.umdl.umich.edu/N02782.0001.001.
5. Bazin H: The ethics of vaccine usage in society: lessons from the past: commentary. *Curr Opin Immunol.* 2001, 13:505-10. 10.1016/S0952-7915(00)00248-X
6. Religious Conviction and the Boston Inoculation Controversy of 1721. (2011). Accessed: June 17, 2018: http://scholarworks.wm.edu/cgi/viewcontent .cgi?referer=https://scholar.google.com/&httpsredir=1&article=1409&context=....
7. 19th-Century Documents Show How Little the Anti-Vaxxers Have Changed. (2014). Accessed: June 17, 2018: http://io9.gizmodo.com/19th-century -documents-show-how-little-the-anti-vaxxers-1658381223.
8. Swales JD: The Leicester anti-vaccination movement. *Lancet.* 1992, 340:1298. 10.1016/0140-6736(92)93006-9
9. Wolfe RM, Sharp LK: Anti-vaccinationists past and present. *BMJ.* 2002, 325:430-32. 10.1136/bmj.325.7361.0
10. Kulenkampff M, Schwartzman JS, Wilson J: Neurological complications of pertussis inoculation. *Arch Dis Child.* 1974, 49:46-49. 10.1136/adc.49.1.46
11. Begg N, White J, Bozoky Z: Media dents confidence in MMR vaccine. *BMJ.* 1998, 316:561. 10.1136/bmj.316.7130.561
12. Gangarosa EJ, Galazka AM, Wolfe CR, et al.: Impact of anti-vaccine movements on pertussis control: the untold story. *Lancet.* 1998, 351:356-61. 10.1016/S0140-6736(97)04334-1
13. Committee on Infectious Diseases: Influenza immunization for all health care personnel: keep it mandatory. *Pediatrics.* 2015, 136:809-18. 10.1542/peds.2015-2922
14. Wakefield AJ, Murch SH, Anthony A, et al.: Ileal-lymphoid-nodular hyperplasia, non-specific colitis, and pervasive developmental disorder in children. *Lancet.* 1998, 351:637-41. 10.1016/S0140-6736(97)11096-0
15. Taylor B, Miller E, Farrington CP, et al.: Autism and measles, mumps, and rubella vaccine: no epidemiological evidence for a causal association. *Lancet.* 1999, 353:2026-29. 10.1016/S0140-6736(99)01239-8
16. Fombonne E, Chakrabarti S: No evidence for a new variant of measles-mumps -rubella-induced autism. *Pediatrics.* 2001, 108:E58. 10.1542/peds.108.4.e58

17. Farrington CP, Miller E, Taylor B: MMR and autism: further evidence against a causal association. *Vaccine.* 2001, 19:3632-35. 10.1016/S0264-410X(01)00097-4

18. DeStefano F, Thompson WW: MMR vaccine and autism: an update of the scientific evidence. *Expert Rev Vaccines.* 2004, 3:19-22. 10.1586/14760584.3.1.19

19. Ferriman A: MP raises new allegations against Andrew Wakefield. *BMJ.* 2004, 328:726. 10.1136/bmj.328.7442.726-a

20. Revealed: MMR Research Scandal. (2004). Accessed: June 17, 2018: http://www.thetimes.co.uk/article/revealed-mmr-research-scandal-7ncfntn8mjq.

21. *Lancet* Retracts "Utterly False" MMR Paper. (2010). Accessed: June 17, 2018: http://www.theguardian.com/society/2010/feb/02/lancet-retracts-mmr-paper.

22. MMR Row Doctor Andrew Wakefield Struck Off Register. (2010). Accessed: June 17, 2018: http://www.theguardian.com/society/2010/may/24/mmr-doctor-andrew-wakefield-struck-off.

23. Murch S: Separating inflammation from speculation in autism. *Lancet.* 2003, 362:1498-99. 10.1016/S0140-6736(03)14699-5

24. McBrien J, Murphy J, Gill D, et al.: Measles outbreak in Dublin, 2000. *Pediatr Infect Dis J.* 2003, 22:580-84. 10.1097/01.inf.0000073059.57867.36

25. UC Research: Vaccinations of US Children Declined after Publication of Now-Refuted Autism Risk. (2012). Accessed: June 17, 2018: http://www.uc.edu/news/NR.aspx?id=15881.

26. Asaria P, MacMahon E: Measles in the United Kingdom: can we eradicate it by 2010? *BMJ.* 2006, 333:890-5. 10.1136/bmj.38989.445845.7C

27. Godlee F, Smith J, Marcovitch H: Wakefield's article linking MMR vaccine and autism was fraudulent. *BMJ.* 2011, 342:c7452. 10.1136/bmj.c7452

28. Pepys MB: Science and serendipity. *Clin Med.* 2007, 7:562-78. 10.7861/clinmedicine.7-6-562

29. Antona D, Lévy-Bruhl D, Baudon C, et al.: Measles elimination efforts and 2008–2011 outbreak, France. *Emerg Infect Dis.* 2013, 19:357-64. 10.3201/eid1903.121360

30. Measles Outbreak Hits 127 People in 15 States. (2008). Accessed: June 17, 2018: http://www.reuters.com/article/us-measles-usa-idUSN0943743120080709.

31. US Measles Surge This Year Is Biggest Since 1996. (2011). Accessed: June 17, 2018: http://www.cidrap.umn.edu/news-perspective/2011/05/us-measles-surge-year-biggest-1996.

32. Measles Outbreak Tied to Texas Megachurch Sickens 21. (2015). Accessed: June 17, 2018: http://www.nbcnews.com/healthmain/measles-outbreak-tied-texas-megachurch-sickens-21-8C11009315.

33. Zipprich J, Winter K, Hacker J, et al.: Measles outbreak—California, December 2014–February 2015. MMWR Morb Mortal Wkly Rep. 2015, 64:153-54. https://www.cdc.gov/mmwr/preview/mmwrhtml/mm6406a5.htm.

34. Majumder MS, Cohn EL, Mekaru SR, et al.: Substandard vaccination compliance and the 2015 measles outbreak. *JAMA Pediatr.* 2015, 169:494-95. 10.1001/jamapediatrics.2015.0384

35. California Governor Signs Vaccine Bill That Bans Personal, Religious Exemptions. (2015). Accessed: June 17, 2018: http://www.cnn.com/2015/06/30/health/california-vaccine-bill/index.html.

36. Forkner-Dunn J: Internet-based patient self-care: the next generation of health care delivery. *J Med Internet Res.* 2003, 5:e8. 10.2196/jmir.5.2.e8

37. Ratzan SC: The plural of anecdote is not evidence. *J Health Commun.* 2002, 7:169-70. 10.1080/10810730290088058

38. Keelan J, Pavri-Garcia V, Tomlinson G, Wilson K: YouTube as a source of information on immunization: a content analysis. *JAMA*. 2007, 298:2482-84. 10.1001/jama.298.21.2482

39. Keelan J, Pavri V, Balakrishnan R, et al.: An analysis of the human papilloma virus vaccine debate on MySpace blogs. *Vaccine*. 2010, 28:1535-40. 10.1016/j. vaccine.2009.11.060

40. Seeman N, Ing A, Rizo C: Assessing and responding in real time to online anti-vaccine sentiment during a flu pandemic. *Healthc Q*. 2010, 13:8-15. 10.12927/ hcq.2010.21923

41. Davies P, Chapman S, Leask J: Antivaccination activists on the world wide web. *Arch Dis Child*. 2002, 87:22-25. 10.1136/adc.87.1.22

42. Kata A: Anti-vaccine activists, Web 2.0, and the postmodern paradigm—an overview of tactics and tropes used online by the anti-vaccination movement. *Vaccine*. 2012, 30: 3778-89. 10.1016/j.vaccine.2011.11.112

43. Kortum P, Edwards C, Richards-Kortum R: The impact of inaccurate Internet health information in a secondary school learning environment. *J Med Internet Res*. 2008, 10:e17. 10.2196/jmir.986

44. Betsch C, Renkewitz F, Betsch T, et al.: The influence of vaccine-critical websites on perceiving vaccination risks. *J Health Psychol*. 2010, 15:446-55. 10.1177/1359105309353647

45. Downs JS, de Bruin BW, Fischhoff B: Parents' vaccination comprehension and decisions. *Vaccine*. 2008, 26:1595-607. 10.1016/j.vaccine.2008.01.011

46. Cooper TL: *The Responsible Administrator: An Approach to Ethics for the Administrative Role*, 6th Ed.. Cooper TL (ed): Jossey-Bass, San Francisco; 2012.

47. Wombwell E, Fangman MT, Yoder AK, Spero DL: Religious barriers to measles vaccination. *J Community Health*. 2015 , 40:597-604. 10.1007/s10900-014-9956-1

48. Karim AA, Bhat R: Gelatin alternatives for the food industry: recent developments, challenges and prospects. *Trends Food Sci Tech*. 2008, 19:644-56. 10.1016/j.tifs.2008.08.001

49. Fine P, Eames K, Heymann DL: "Herd immunity": a rough guide. *Clin Infect Dis*. 2011, 52:911-916. 10.1093/cid/cir007

50. Bouton CW: John Stuart Mill: on liberty and history. *West Polit Q*. 1965, 18:569-78.

8

Past Pandemics Led to the First International Disease Control Efforts

Anne-Emanuelle Birn

Anne-Emanuelle Birn is a professor of critical development studies and of social and behavioral health sciences at the University of Toronto, Canada. She served as the Canada Research Chair in International Health from 2003 to 2013.

Before the rise of nation-states and the possibility of governmental actions to control the spread of infectious diseases, the first disease control efforts emerged as a result of the Justinian Plague and the Black Death of the Middle Ages. City-states, quarantine boards, hospitals, religious orders, and printers are counted among those who helped to establish improved hygienic safeguards and processes. By the eighteenth century and the rise of urban centers, new sanitation measures stood a fighting chance against deadly diseases.

What do we think of when we hear the word "plague"? Red crosses on boarded-up doors? Deserted medieval villages? Or maybe the horror film–esque cloak and mask of a plague doctor?

Unsurprisingly, the history of plague and its impact on health regulation is more complex and far-reaching than many assume. This extract from the *Textbook of Global Health* looks at the medical

"How Did the Plague Impact Health Regulation?" by Anne-Emanuelle Birn, Oxford University Press, March 20, 2018. Reprinted by permission.

and environmental legacy of pandemics, which range from the Plague of Justinian, to the infamous Black Death and beyond.

For the most part, scientific ideas, technologies, and practices in medieval Europe trailed those of other societies, particularly in the Islamic world, where influential advances were made in such areas as astronomy, surgery, theories of disease-transmission, mind-body connections, and medical institutions. European healing involved a combination of local wisdom (e.g., knowledge of medicinal herbs passed down from generation to generation and among lay practitioners, including midwives who apprenticed with other wise women) and a hierarchy of town-based practitioners, such as apothecaries, barber-surgeons, and university-trained physicians.

It was during the Middle Ages that hospitals and religious orders dedicated to healing were established in Europe, partly to care for crusaders returning from Church-sanctioned military campaigns to recapture Palestine from Muslim control. Some institutions, such as St. Bartholomew's in London, founded in 1123, still function today, as does Santa Maria Nuova in Florence. From about the 13th century on, secular hospitals were also founded in many larger European cities, though there was continued importance of the complementary role of the healing of the body and the healing of the soul.

Other changes were afoot that would test sanitary localism and Europe's backwardness. As rival leaders fought for land and power (needing ever greater resources for these exploits), and merchants became interested in the riches and resources of faraway places, travel and commerce gradually increased, with microbes as companions. The congested towns of late medieval Europe were typified by poor sanitation and hygiene in comparison to some contemporary civilizations elsewhere, such as the Aztec Empire, and thus became loci of epidemic disease.

Plague is among the earliest documented pandemics, with two great outbreaks bracketing the Middle Ages. The first, known as the Plague of Justinian, struck in 542 CE, decimating populations throughout Eurasia. The second pandemic began with the Black

Death in 1347 and lasted until the late 17th century. It was the most destructive epidemic in the history of humankind, which resulted in an estimated 100 million deaths (almost one quarter of the world's population, especially striking Asia, Europe, and the Middle East).

Surmised to have originated in wild rodents (probably in Central Asia), whose habitats were disrupted by a mix of human invasion, expansion of farming lands, and new trading patterns, what became known as the Black Death traveled by land and water along the Silk Road. It reached the Black Sea in 1346. By 1348 it had spread northward to Russia, westward to Europe, eastward toward China, and south-westward to the Middle East.

Although its cause was unknown, plague's suspected communicability led to the earliest attempts at international disease control. In 1348, believing that plague was introduced via ships, the city-state of Venice adopted a 40-day detention period for entering vessels (a policy soon copied by Genoa, Marseille, and other major ports) after which the disease was believed to remit. This practice of quarantine—from the Italian word for forty—was minimally effective in stopping plague. Quarantine's stricter counterpart, the cordon sanitaire—a protective geographic belt barring exit of people or goods from cities or entire regions—would also be used frequently in succeeding centuries. In 1423 Venice established the first lazaretto, a quarantine station to hold and disinfect humans and cargo. Its island location was emulated by other cities across the world.

Because the Black Death's initial appearance preceded the formation of nation-states, sanitary efforts in the 14th century were adopted and implemented by municipal authorities with little coordination. While word of disease spread through travelers, initially there was no official system of notification or cooperation between city-states. However, by the 15th century many Italian towns and cities established plague boards, sometimes made into permanent public health boards, charged with imposing the necessary measures at times of outbreak. This precursor to international health authority, though local, rapidly developed a cooperative dimension through frequent correspondence between the plague boards.

Over time, new ideas evolved around plague's communicability, justifying ever-stricter quarantine measures. In 1546, the Veronese physician-scholar Girolamo Fracastoro revived ancient notions of contagion in his tract on plague transmission, theorizing that "seeds of disease" could be spread either through direct contact or by dissemination into the atmosphere.

Though the virulence of plague lessened somewhat in the 15th century, subsequent visitations worsened. In 1630–1631, plague killed one quarter of the population in Bologna, one third in Venice, almost half in Milan, and almost two-thirds in Verona. A scant generation later, half of the inhabitants of Rome, Naples, and Genoa succumbed to the plague of 1656–1657.

Plague, of course, was not the only deadly or epidemic ailment of the Middle Ages and early modern period. Smallpox, diphtheria, measles, influenza, tuberculosis, scabies, erysipelas, anthrax, trachoma, leprosy, and nutritional deficiencies were also rife. Less familiar today, mass hysteria in a climate of superstition led to outbreaks of dancing mania (St. Vitus Dance). Ergotism, arising from fungal contamination of rye, killed or disabled large numbers of people in dozens of epidemics between the 9th and 15th centuries.

Spurred on by more stringent sanitary enforcement during plague years, concepts of cleanliness and sanitation gradually took hold in Europe's cities. Through increasingly forceful legislation and public awareness, announced via the printing press (c. 1440) and town criers, urban centers began to approach the hygienic standards reached by the Roman Empire more than a millennium earlier. Influenced by neo-Hippocratic ideas on the link between health and "airs, waters and places," health boards and many local governments took on more rigorous control of street cleaning, disposal of dead bodies and carcasses, public baths, and water maintenance. By the 18th century, cities began to employ, fitfully, a new environmental engineering approach to epidemic disease, which emphasized preventive actions including improved ventilation, drainage of stagnant water, street cleaning, reinternment, cleaner wells, fumigation, and the burial of garbage.

Even before the plague fully retreated, a new economic system began to develop that would irrevocably shape worldwide patterns of disease and eventually lead to international health measures and institutions.

9

The Connection Between Slavery and the First Yellow Fever Pandemic

Billy G. Smith

Billy G. Smith is a professor in the Department of History, Philosophy, and Religious Studies at Montana State University in Bozeman, Montana. He is the author of Ship of Death: The Voyage That Changed the Atlantic World.

In 1792, a group of anti-slavery British citizens set out to hire rather than enslave Africans. But once in West Africa, where they hoped to establish a colony, they contracted yellow fever. Those who survived tried to return to Britain but ended up in the Caribbean. From there, other ships traveled to Philadelphia, bringing yellow fever with them. This pandemic affected the US government and even motivated the decision to move the nation's capital from Philadelphia to Washington, DC. Moreover, the pandemic put in place the myth that African Americans had immunity to the disease, which only served to promote racial prejudices in the years to come.

Bird flu, SARS, Marburg, Ebola, HIV, West Nile Fever. One of these diseases, or another, that spread from animals and mosquitoes to humans may soon kill most people on the planet. More likely, the great majority of us will survive such a world-wide pandemic, and even now we have a heightened awareness that another one may be on the horizon. This blog focuses on

"The First Yellow Fever Pandemic: Slavery and Its Consequences," by Billy G. Smith, the New York Academy of Medicine, October 15, 2018. Reprinted by permission of the author.

these issues in the past, outlining a virtually unknown voyage of death and disease that transformed the communities and nations bordering the Atlantic Ocean (what historians now refer to as the Atlantic World). It traces the journey of a sailing ship that inadvertently instigated an epidemiological tragedy, thereby transforming North America, Europe, Africa, and the Caribbean islands. This ship helped to create the first yellow fever pandemic.

In 1792, the *Hankey* and two other ships carried nearly three hundred idealistic antislavery British radicals to Bolama, an island off the coast of West Africa, where they hoped to establish a colony designed to undermine the Atlantic slave trade by hiring rather than enslaving Africans. Poor planning and tropical diseases, especially a particularly virulent strain of yellow fever likely contracted from the island's numerous monkeys (through a mosquito vector), decimated the colonists and turned the enterprise into a tragic farce.

In early 1793, after most colonists had died and survivors had met resistance from the indigenous Bijagos for invading their lands, the *Hankey* attempted to return to Britain. Disease-ridden, lacking healthy sailors, and fearing interception by hostile French ships, the colonists caught the trade winds to Grenada. They and the mosquitoes in the water barrels spread yellow fever in that port and, very soon, throughout the West Indies. This was only a few months before the British arrived to quell the slave rebellion in St. Domingue (now Haiti). The British and subsequently the French military had their troops decimated by the disease—one reason why the slave revolution succeeded. The crushing defeat in the Caribbean helped convince Napoleon to sell the vast Louisiana territory to the United States. He turned eastward to expand his empire, altering the future of Europe and the Americas.

A few months after the *Hankey* arrived in the West Indies, commercial and refugee ships carried passengers and mosquitoes infected with yellow fever to Philadelphia, the nation's capital during the 1790s. The resulting epidemic killed five thousand people and forced tens of thousands of residents, including George

Washington, Thomas Jefferson, and other prominent federal government leaders, to flee for their lives. The state, city, and federal government all collapsed, leaving it to individual citizens to save the nation's capital. Meanwhile, doctors fiercely debated whether "Bulama fever" (as many called it) was a "new" disease or a more virulent strain of yellow fever common in the West Indies. Physicians like the noted Benjamin Rush fiercely debated the causes of and treatment for the disease. They mostly bled and purged their patients, at times causing more harm than good because of the rudimentary state of medicine.

Among those who stepped forward to aid people and save the city were members of the newly emerging community of free African Americans. Led by Absalom Jones, Richard Allen, and Anne Saville, black Philadelphians volunteered to nurse the sick and bury the dead—both dangerous undertakings at the time. Many African Americans and physicians, exposed to yellow-fever infected mosquitoes, made the ultimate sacrifice as both groups died in disproportionately high numbers. When a newspaper editor subsequently maligned black people for their efforts, Jones and Allen wrote a vigorous response—among the first publications by African Americans in the new nation.

During the ensuing decade, yellow fever went global, afflicting every port city in the new nation on an annual basis. Epidemics also occurred in metropolitan areas throughout the Atlantic World, including North and South America, the Caribbean, southern Europe, and Africa. Among other consequences, this disaster encouraged Americans to fear cities as hubs of death. The future of the United States, as Thomas Jefferson argued, would be rural areas populated by yeomen farmers rather than the people in teeming metropolises. The epidemics also helped solidify the decision of leaders of the new nation to move its capital to Washington, D.C., and away from the high mortality associated with Philadelphia.

After the *Hankey* finally limped home to Britain, its crew was taken into service in the Royal Navy; few of them survived long. More importantly, the image of Africa as the "white man's graveyard" became even more established in Britain and France, thereby providing a partially protective barrier for Africa from European invasion until the advent of tropical medicine. The "Bulama fever" plagued the Atlantic World for the next half century, appearing in epidemic form from Spain to Africa to North and South America. The origins and treatment of the disease drew intense debates as medical treatment became highly politicized, and the incorrect idea that Africans enjoyed immunity to yellow fever became an important part of the scientific justification of racism in the early nineteenth century.

10

Fear Motivated a Useless Flu Immunization Campaign in 1976

Joan Trossman Bien

Joan Trossman Bien is a Los Angeles–based freelance journalist whose work focuses on medical and mental health issues.

In 1976, five people at Fort Dix in New Jersey fell sick from the swine flu, and one soldier died. This stirred up memories of the deadly flu pandemic of 1918. President Gerald Ford, who came into office without executive experience as a result of President Richard Nixon's resignation, called for a nationwide immunization program. Experts debated the efficacy of such a program, and many who tried to receive immunization ended up getting the incorrect vaccine. In the end, the program was a complete failure, but luckily a pandemic never emerged from an isolated outbreak. Still, fears have remained of an influenza pandemic comparable to the 1918 pandemic.

America was one raw nerve. An unpopular Republican president had left office, leaving behind an unpopular war to wind down. Democrats now ruled both houses of Congress. The sitting president, a Midwesterner whose ascendancy had been historic, came in without executive experience. The country was deeply divided among itself and cynical distrust of government and corporations alike was rampant. It was 1976.

"The Swine Flu Vaccine: 1976 Casts a Giant Shadow," by Joan Trossman Bien, the Social Justice Foundation, June 14, 2017. Reprinted by permission.

It had been 58 years since the 1918 flu pandemic, called the Spanish flu because Spain's open reporting on the flu's ravages made it seem more awful than in more censored nations. Survivors of the deadly influenza often censored their own recollections, so the pandemic took a backseat to many of the 20th century's other tragedies. Then an outbreak of swine flu at Fort Dix, N.J., sickened five and on Feb. 6, 1976, one soldier died, and global health officials recalled just how awful a flu can be.

Prologue

March 1918 was a difficult time for the nation. America had waded into the European nightmare of the Great War. Gripped by a patriotic fever, civilians endured food rationing and press censorship. When the call went out for medical personnel to support the troops, doctors and nurses answered in droves, leaving the home front with an inexperienced and depleted medical community.

On March 4, the flu broke out at Fort Riley, Kan. The illness was referred to as the "three-day fever," and as the soldiers left Kansas for Europe, this fever went with them. The afflicted were often hale and young—many older Americans still carried some immunity to it as a holdover from the 1889–90 Russian flu.

The virus thrived in the trenches and the putrid conditions troops were forced to endure. Many of the soldiers' lungs had been devastated by mustard gas. Casualties were jammed into temporary military hospitals that defied attempts at any meaningful hygiene practices.

In August 1918, a far more virulent form of the virus emerged simultaneously in Brest in France, Freetown in South Africa and in Boston. The appearance of this mutated influenza was so sudden and so deadly that some speculated it was a German biological weapon.

As the troops returned home on crowded ships and trains, they again brought the virus with them. On Nov. 11, 1918, Americans celebrated the end of the war and Armistice Day by attending large parties and parades. Although nearly 200,000 had perished during the month of October, the flu appeared to have peaked. But the public gatherings, from a public health view, poured gasoline onto a dying ember. The flu exploded across the country in another wave, killing young, healthy adults at 20 times the rate of previous influenzas.

Death by Spanish flu was particularly hideous. It often attacked and killed within hours, although secondary infections contributed significantly to the spiking mortality rates. The flu had morphed into a raging hemorrhagic virus. Once cyanosis set in, the patient's face would turn bluish-grey, their lungs filled with bloody froth and the edema slowly suffocated them as they gasped for air. Blood pouring from a victim's nose and mouth, ears and eyes became the hallmarks of this pandemic.

Fame and wealth offered no protection. Sigmund Freud's daughter, Sophie, died from influenza as did the daughter of Buffalo Bill Cody. William Randolph Hearst's mother died as did Donald Trump's grandfather and the author of "Cyrano de Bergerac," Edmond Rostand.

President Woodrow Wilson fell ill during the negotiations of the Treaty of Versailles and recovered, as did future president Franklin D. Roosevelt. British Prime Minister David Lloyd George, artist Georgia O'Keeffe, author Katherine Anne Porter, Gen. John J. Pershing, and visionary Walt Disney all survived the flu.

The Spanish flu killed 675,000 Americans, many times more than died in the war. When it was over, the lifespan of Americans had been shortened by 12 years.

The world had never seen a devastating holocaust of disease like the 1918–1919 influenza. It killed so swiftly, it is estimated some 25 million died in the pandemic's first 25 weeks, as many as died in Europe's Black Plague and more than the dead from the Great War's battlefields. Approximately half of the world's population had been infected. Recent estimates of the flu's deadly toll range from at least 50 million up to 100 million.

Act I

The Fredericksburg, Va., *Free-Lance Star* on Feb. 20, 1976, picked up the Associated Press story about the swine flu death. The headline blared "Killer Flu Back On Scene: No Immediate Cause for Alarm."

The story read, "The Center for Disease Control has reported an outbreak of influenza in humans similar to a virus found in swine—and recalling the flu of a half-century ago..."

The *Los Angeles Times* ran a brief update from AP on Feb. 25, 1976. "Blood tests on 241 GIs 'showed evidence' that 63 may have contracted and recovered from a swine-type variation of Influenza A, the Army said Tuesday. An Army spokesman said that in some of the 63 men, the virus apparently created antibodies that helped dispel the disease. He said all of the men had been in recent contact with five soldiers who were stricken with swine flu. One of the five died."

The Washington Post on March 24 wrote that President Gerald Ford was considering a flu immunization program that would be the largest in this country's history. "Government experts, backed by the recommendations of two advisory committees, decided that all 215 million Americans should receive protection against the swine flu....Most health experts believe that the new type of swine flu will spread around the country next winter."

The publicity machine of the federal government was gearing up with the full cooperation of the press.

On March 30, the Toledo (Ohio) *Blade* played down the flu danger. A microbiologist at the Mayo Clinic was quoted saying the same swine flu virus that was so worrisome to the government had been isolated from a cancer victim. The scientist concluded that this virus may have been "occurring undetected for years in America without causing the epidemic officials now fear."

On the same day, the AP reported the government line: "Nobody knows for certain whether there will be a flu outbreak in the US this coming winter, but the risks are too high to gamble on doing nothing, officials said as the medical drama unfolded."

The director of Public Citizen's Health Group, Dr. Sidney M. Wolfe, sounded a warning of possible serious side effects from the vaccine. On April 11, he wrote an essay in the *Los Angeles Times* in which he cast doubt on the similarity between the one case of swine flu at Fort Dix and the 1918 pandemic.

Most worrying to Wolfe was a request by one of the four pharmaceutical manufacturers for the federal government to relax standards for testing the toxicity of the vaccine in order to ensure an adequate supply. He said now the risk of illness had switched to the vaccine itself.

Citing a complete absence of the reappearance of the swine flu in the two months since the death of the one soldier at Ft. Dix, Wolfe said, "Unless there is a real need and unless the preventive measure is effective and safe, relative to the disease it seeks to prevent, the prevention or 'cure' may be worse than the disease."

A new wrinkle in the government mass immunization plans appeared on April 12 in the *Los Angeles Times*. The president of the Pharmaceutical Manufacturers Association explained that since the industry had not been able to get statutory immunity in the case of possible adverse reactions to the vaccine, the companies now were simply refusing to make it. "The planned mass immunization against the swine flu next fall may be jeopardized by a Senate committee's recommendation that vaccine makers be liable for any adverse reactions," he said.

Two weeks later, in its April 26 issue, *Time* magazine wrote that the vaccine makers had been granted their request by the federal government to lower the manufacturing standards. "It has obliged them by dropping one of its new mandatory measurements for impurities in vaccines."

Polio vaccine developer Dr. Albert Sabin voiced second thoughts about the vaccination program. The *Los Angeles Times* on May 18 reported on an address that Sabin had recently given at the College of Pharmacy at the University of Toledo. "In my own mind now I am wondering very seriously if it would not be very prudent to make as much vaccine as possible and not use it until there is evidence this virus is spreading in the United States," he was quoted. Sabin was concerned that if the virus returned, an early vaccination might not provide immunity long enough.

The *Los Angeles Times* ran a UPI story on May 19 comparing the 1918 flu pandemic and the 1976 swine flu. It said the 1918 Spanish flu first occurred at a US Army camp, as did the one case of swine flu in 1976. It mentioned that the 1918 flu killed more than 10 times as many Americans as died in World War I, with 852 deaths occurring in New York City in one day. The article said the 1918 flu virus simply disappeared at the end of the pandemic and scientists had been at a loss to explain where it went or whether it would ever reappear.

On June 3, a UPI story in *Ellensburg* (Wash.) *Daily Record* stated that one of the four companies making the vaccine, Parke-Davis, had made a huge error. Among the 2.6 million doses that it had manufactured, an unknown number had been based on a similar but different flu virus. "Some human test subjects were given the wrong vaccine in the clinical trials which began in April and have covered 3,200 volunteers, 600 of them children."

The immunization program appeared to be headed for complete failure on June 16 when the *Spokesman-Review* out of Spokane, Wash., reported that two of the four manufacturers no longer had liability insurance coverage for the vaccine and that a third firm was about to lose its insurance.

What might have been the death knell for the program occurred June 29. The *St. Petersburg Times* reported that based on the clinical trials of 5,000 people, Sabin had recommended the plan should be scrapped. The studies had shown that older people were already armed with antibodies to the swine flu, and there wasn't enough vaccine to provide so-called "herd immunity" in the rest of the populace.

On July 2, an AP story in the *Free-Lance Star* reported that in light of the vaccine makers' inability to obtain liability insurance, the only option would be for the federal government to indemnify those companies, an idea that was not getting support in Washington. "A House Health subcommittee...refused to consider an administration bill that would have freed manufacturers of most liability in the massive inoculation program and would have put the responsibility on the government."

The grand plan to ward off a deadly influenza virus pandemic through a massive vaccination program had all but collapsed.

Act II

In July, Americans celebrating the nation's 200th birthday saw large groups gather in patriotic fervor, particularly in Philadelphia. But a mysterious illness at a veterans' gathering in that city breathed a new spark into the near-extinguished immunization plan: Men present earlier at an American Legion convention suddenly became ill; some died within days of the first symptoms.

On July 23, Michigan's *Ludington Daily News* printed a UPI story, "The medical mystery over the American Legion killer disease deepened today. Dreaded swine flu has become less likely and bacteria was eliminated from the list of possible causes of the illness that killed 22 persons and hospitalized scores more."

Still, newspapers began to refer to this new and deadly illness as a "flu-like" disease. In a *Los Angeles Times* story on Aug. 3, the Pennsylvania health secretary was asked if it could be swine flu. "That's a possibility," he said.

A spokesman for that same department added, "It doesn't seem to be related to food poisoning....They have flu symptoms. It looks like flu."

The article went on to quote the personal physician of a 60-year-old man who died July 26: "I've had several influenza deaths over the last 30 years, and there are some influenza symptoms here. First you get a cold, and the next thing you know you're sicker than hell, and the next thing you're dead."

On August 17, the *Los Angeles Times* reported the death toll was still climbing. A total of 26 people—all at the American Legion convention—had died within a few weeks.

What would turn out to be a new and novel illness called "Legionnaires' Disease" revived the lifeless government immunization program. The August 23 issue of *Time* magazine reported the lopsided vote in Congress to shoulder all liability for the swine flu vaccination program.

Scrutiny of the vaccine's possible side effects was intense. The *Los Angeles Times* reported on Oct. 14 that the CDC unwaveringly continued to support the program, saying, "There is no evidence that the program should be curtailed in any way," even after the post-vaccination deaths of 24 elderly people. The bottom of the article noted, "The average age of those who died was 72.1, and all but one had a history of heart disease."

Also on Oct. 14, newspapers reported President Ford publicly receiving his own vaccination in an effort to calm concerns about the vaccine.

On Oct. 26, the *Los Angeles Times* ran a feature referencing the 1918 flu. Elderly people standing in line to receive their vaccinations recalled what it had actually been like to live through the pandemic. They said they were disgusted that younger people were more afraid of the vaccine than they were of the flu. Remembering the horrors of it, one woman said, "Oh, it's just terrible, dreadful. You get a sore throat, high fever, vomiting, and finally you can't breathe anymore at all. It's the worst way to watch someone die."

On the first day that swine flu shots were available to the general public, only 5,030 people in Los Angeles County showed up to receive the immunization.

On Dec. 15, a new reason to skip the vaccine made headlines. The *St. Petersburg Times* combined AP and UPI reports and wrote, "Federal health officials said...they are investigating reports that at least 30 persons who received swine flu shots later developed a temporary paralysis. The national CDC said it picked up reports of the paralysis, known as Guillain-Barre syndrome, through its own extensive flu surveillance network." The syndrome's cause is unknown but the onset is often associated with infections, surgery, influenza and vaccines.

On Dec. 16, 1976, the federal government shut down the mass swine flu immunization program. A statistical association between the vaccine and the syndrome had been calculated by the CDC.

Guillain-Barre is extremely rare, usually affecting one person in 100,000. In the 1976 swine flu immunization program, 48 million Americans were vaccinated; Guillain-Barre infected 532 people and 25 died.

Epilogue

As of November 2009, more than 1,000 Americans had died from the current H1N1 influenza, with 48 states reporting this flu. The flu season typically runs from October through March.

Whether the current strain of H1N1, still considered to be mild, will mutate into a more virulent form in another wave, as did the 1918 flu pandemic, remains to be seen.

In 1976, one person died from the swine flu. That strain quickly faded away and has not reappeared. To say that more people died from the vaccine than from the flu is not a universal truth but a highly unusual set of facts. Had the swine flu reappeared, the historic record on the value of the vaccinations would have been different.

11

How to Lie with Statistics: The Case of HIV/AIDS in Southern Africa

Ernest Harsch

Ernest Harsch is a researcher with Columbia University's Institute of African Studies. He worked on African issues at the United Nations for more than twenty years. There he served as managing editor of the journal Africa Renewal.

Statistics reported from rural areas in particular may not be reliable, and this frequently causes debate among expert organizations. Although statistics indicated that AIDS deaths declined in the first decade of the new millennium, epidemic cases still persisted, especially in southern Africa, where a third of those afflicted with the disease lived. Vigilance still must be taken worldwide. AIDS has long-lasting effects that require monitoring, and regardless of what the statistics imply, ample resources are required to continue treatment and eradication measures.

For the first time since the AIDS pandemic was identified a quarter-century ago, "we are seeing a decline in global AIDS deaths," reports Dr. Kevin De Cock, director of AIDS at the World Health Organization (WHO). Revised figures released by WHO and the Joint UN Programme on HIV/AIDS (UNAIDS) also show that new infections from HIV, the virus that causes the disease, have begun to fall as well.

Citing more accurate data-collection methods, the AIDS Epidemic Update 2007, released jointly by UNAIDS and WHO in November, estimates that there are about 33.2 million people worldwide living with HIV, compared with the figure of 39.5 million the two institutions had released the year before. The change in the number of people living with HIV was not an actual decline, the Update hastened to add, but a statistical revision of estimates after detailed national surveys in about 30 countries demonstrated that earlier totals were too high.

The revision generated considerable controversy, with some independent AIDS experts arguing that the data should have been adjusted earlier. But all agree that the newer, more accurate figures have brought into the open an important shift in the epidemic's progression, one that was not apparent with the older statistics.

In adjusting their overall estimates retroactively, to previous years, the two UN institutions revealed some positive trends over time. First, new infections with HIV were likely to have peaked in the late 1990s, when more than 3 million people became newly infected annually. The revised estimates indicate that this total has actually been declining since then, to some 2.5 million newly infected in 2007. Second, the number of annual deaths from AIDS has also started to fall, from a high point of around 2.4 million in 2005 to about 2.1 million in 2007.

To an extent, these changing trends reflect some of the first significant successes in AIDS-prevention efforts. In a number of countries, according to national survey results, young people are engaging in less risky sexual behaviour, whether by using protective condoms or by having fewer or no partners. The report cites evidence of such behavioural changes in Botswana, Cameroon, Kenya, Malawi, Togo, Zambia, Zimbabwe and a few other countries.

"Real Nightmares" in Africa

Neither the shift in the disease's overall trend nor the revision in the estimates has changed one glaring fact: sub-Saharan Africa remains the epicentre of the global malady. Of all those living with HIV, about 22.5 million, or 68 percent of the world's total, are in sub-Saharan Africa. The region accounts for the same percentage of people newly infected with the virus, as well as 76 percent of those who die of AIDS annually.

"AIDS continues to be the single largest cause of mortality in sub-Saharan Africa," says the report. Moreover, in contrast to other world regions, women and children are far more vulnerable to the disease in sub-Saharan Africa. Of those Africans living with HIV, 61 percent are women, while fully 90 percent of all HIV-positive children in the world are in sub-Saharan Africa.

Within the continent, Southern Africa is by far the most afflicted, accounting for around a third of all new HIV infections globally and about a third of people living with HIV. In eight countries—Botswana, Lesotho, Mozambique, Namibia, South Africa, Swaziland, Zambia and Zimbabwe—national adult HIV-prevalence rates exceed 15 percent. South Africa leads the world in the number of people infected with HIV.

Southern African countries, says Daniel Halperin, an AIDS expert at the US's Harvard School of Public Health, are continuing to experience "real nightmares." Whatever else the revision in the overall AIDS figures may show, he adds, "this doesn't mean the epidemic is going away."

Statistical Refinements

In poor, largely rural countries with weak health systems and limited ability to collect data, measuring the extent of an infectious disease is always difficult, notes Dr. Paul De Lay, a UNAIDS director. "The challenge is equally true for TB, polio and childhood diarrhoea."

In the case of HIV/AIDS, earlier estimates were based mainly on information collected on young women visiting public health clinics either because they were pregnant or because they feared they had been infected. Those results were then extrapolated to the rest of the population to come up with estimated national infection rates. But over time experts realized that data from urban clinics were skewed: they gave too much statistical weight to sex workers, drug users and people with multiple partners, relative to other sectors of the population.

As donor countries gradually began providing more funds to combat the disease, some of those resources were allocated for more scientifically designed national surveys, at a cost of $2–3 million per country. Across the board, the surveys showed that the scale of the epidemic was somewhat less than previously thought.

According to UNAIDS, analyses of national survey results in India in July reduced estimates of the number of people living with HIV in that country by more than half, from 5.7 million people to 2.5 million, a revision that accounted for half of the decline in the global estimate. Much of the remaining adjustment, reports UNAIDS, came from revised estimates for several African countries, including Angola, Kenya, Mozambique, Nigeria and Zimbabwe.

Some independent AIDS researchers had been arguing for several years that the UN's earlier estimates were too high, and complain that their arguments were ignored. A few charged that the figures were consciously exaggerated as part of a strategy to raise international alarm about the disease and prompt donors to release more funds. Dr. De Lay regards such accusations as "absurd." It would be "technically impossible" for UNAIDS "to somehow rig the numbers," he says, since they are gathered by national health ministries and reviewed by many experts inside and outside the UN system.

No Time for Complacency

Whether the numbers are going up or down, there should be no complacency, UNAIDS and other experts warn. There is still no cure for AIDS, Dr. De Lay points out. Moreover, in a number of countries that had previously made progress in reducing infection rates, but in which anti-AIDS programmes have diminished, "we are seeing a return of the epidemic," he notes. The *Update* reports that prevalence rates are rising again in the US, the UK and Germany—as well as in Uganda, which once was hailed for its success in bringing down HIV rates.

Nor should the international community slacken its own efforts, argue AIDS advocates. Current international spending, at around $10 billion annually, continues to fall short of actual needs. "There's still a huge epidemic out there that still needs huge resources to win the battle," says Paul Zeitz, executive director of the Global AIDS Alliance, an international non-governmental group headquartered in Washington, DC.

UNAIDS and WHO are planning to issue a report in 2008 on financing the global campaign against AIDS. It is possible, says Dr. De Lay, that projected treatment costs, such as for providing anti-retroviral medicines to people with full-blown AIDS, will be about 5 percent less in 2010 than previously estimated. But that total will still be around $38 billion—far higher than current AIDS financing.

"We have to recognize the very long-term nature of the HIV pandemic," says Dr. De Cock. "We're facing decades of this problem." Of those currently infected, "some of them require treatment now, and all of them will in time. The qualitative implications have changed very little."

12

Animal Health Affects Human Health: The Case of Ebola

Arinjay Banerjee, Colin Brown, and Grant Hill-Cawthorne

Arinjay Banerjee is a postdoctoral research fellow at McMaster University in Canada. Colin Brown is the Infectious Disease Lead for the King's Sierra Leone Partnership, King's College, London. Grant Hill-Cawthorne is a senior lecturer in communicable disease epidemiology at the University of Sydney in Australia.

The Ebola virus originated in animals and has proven to be deadly to humans through outbreak, epidemic, and pandemic occurrences. Organizations such as the World Health Organization must coordinate efforts with the Food and Agriculture Organization to recognize the importance of animal health to human health. Only by analyzing how animals and humans interact within the environment can we strike a preemptive blow against the deadly emergence and spread of this virus.

R ight now the World Health Organization (WHO) is holding its annual World Health Assembly (WHA). At this time last year, Ebola Virus Disease (EVD) was rapidly spreading through West Africa, and the outbreak is rightly a major item on this year's assembly agenda. Attention will be paid to the decisions made in response to the outbreak and what this tells us about how best to respond to the next one, including for advance preparation and early warning.

WHO Director-General Margaret Chan has already outlined her plans for a US$100 million contingency fund to support emergency response capacity in future outbreaks. This is welcome news.

The EVD outbreak in West Africa demonstrates how important the interaction between human and animal health is. It is a zoonotic infection, which means it originated in animals (bats, in this case) before spreading into humans. So, alongside better strategies to respond to outbreaks in human populations, we also need to have a stronger focus on disease surveillance in animals to identify infectious diseases before they pose a risk to human health.

One Health, a discipline through which we examine how the interactions of humans, animals and the environment come together to allow an infectious threat to arise, develop and become a sustained outbreak, could have informed a better preemptive response to the virus.

How Did Ebola Become a Major Outbreak?

Ebola causes harmless, asymptomatic infection in bats. It took one encounter (or entry cause) for the virus to spill into humans. After that initial encounter, the disease was able to spread through communities in West Africa because of limited public health infrastructure. The regional population is highly connected, which led to an exponential increase in cases. There was also a lack of diagnostics for other infectious diseases. Unfortunately, the global community was slow to take action.

In the affected areas, there was a lack of awareness about EVD and its transmission, which allowed the spread of disease. This emphasizes the need for education and communication in the community that involve local leaders as well.

Responding to the Outbreak

When it became clear that EVD had the potential to go from a severe regional outbreak to a pandemic, interdisciplinary teams arrived to help the overwhelmed domestic healthcare system control the epidemic.

Doctors Without Borders (MSF) was the first to highlight that this was an unprecedented outbreak, as early as March 2014, following the first reporting of the outbreak. Local development partners such as King's Sierra Leone Partnership, an international health link through King's College London, took on leadership roles in outbreak control in partnership with national government response.

But it was only in the latter part of the outbreak that epidemiologists and wildlife scientists began assisting in identifying the potential source of the outbreak—possibly bats roosting inside a hollow tree in Meliandou, Guinea.

One Health wasn't applied in the early stages of the outbreak to assess the likelihood of multiple entry points into the human population, and no pre-outbreak surveillance had been undertaken in West Africa.

The Social Context of the Ebola Outbreak

The cultural setting of West Africa has been much discussed, but hinders the understanding of this outbreak by ignoring the political and economic global forces that left West Africa vulnerable.

Long-standing cultural practices, such as washing deceased relatives, further spread the disease. Early and targeted engagement with local community leaders about infection control should be a key component of future outbreak control.

However, simply focusing on human public health isn't enough when it comes to a zoonotic infection. We also need to focus on how an outbreak like this can affect animal populations. The debate on the Ebola response has focused nearly entirely on human fatalities, ignoring the potentially far-reaching and largely undocumented impact on nonhuman primates.

And discussions focused on banning bushmeat ignore human economic concerns and the critically endangered nature of at-risk animal populations being further decimated by EVD in West Africa.

Prediction and Surveillance

Prediction, or at the very least understanding, of possible threats should be a key goal of future risk reduction strategies, to ensure we prevent another "Black Swan": an unexpected major event that comes as a complete surprise, "rationalized after the fact with the benefit of hindsight."

For infectious diseases, prediction rests on strong disease surveillance in both human and animal populations. We could have predicted West Africa was susceptible to EVD, but such surveillance doesn't currently form any of the decision-making processes that are used globally.

The main international treaty underpinning health security, the International Health Regulations (2005) (IHR 2005), requires the 195 member states of the WHO to have in place "core capacity requirements for surveillance and response to events."

By the initial deadline of 2012, only 42 countries had met their core capacity requirements. By the end of June 2014, four months into the Ebola outbreak, only a further 21 met these requirements. Fewer than one-third of the WHO member states have declared their compliance with IHR 2005. Efforts to help poorer nations to achieve this have not been forthcoming. This means that the majority of member states still lack adequate human disease surveillance.

However, complying with IHR 2005 does not guarantee that countries are able to detect emerging zoonotic diseases. The checklist for monitoring progress toward IHR core capacities does not include animal or wildlife disease surveillance.

The WHA 2015 has focused on renewed calls to strengthen human disease surveillance. But as an international community, we need to consider early combined surveillance of both humans and animals. There should no longer be a complete division between ministries of health and wildlife agencies.

The goals of the WHO in curbing the spread of the infectious disease must align with those of the World Organization for Animal Health and Food and Agriculture Organization of the United Nations to ensure that infectious disease threats are targeted from their transmission from animals to humans through to managing their quarantine and public health control.

The $100 million contingency fund is a welcome step in the right direction. But now international aid needs to focus on developing public health systems that are robust, effective and cross-species. Disregard of animal well-being comes at our own cost.

13

Outbreaks Among the Poor Go Unnoticed and Unreported

Ben Oppenheim and Gavin Yamey

Ben Oppenheim is a senior fellow and visiting scholar at the New York University Center on International Cooperation. Gavin Yamey is a professor of the practice at the Duke University Sanford School of Public Policy and an associate of the Duke Initiative for Science and Society.

As early as 1848, researchers established that the poor were harder hit by epidemics and pandemics than the rest of the population. Through a study of pandemics and their increased likelihood arising from a combination of environmental, ecological, and social factors, monitoring appears as a vital step in containing the spread. But among the poor, outbreaks are likely to go unreported, since poverty-stricken areas lack trained personnel and other resources. A four-point plan can help rectify the situation and provide assistance to these areas while also restricting the spread of disease.

When epidemics or pandemics hit, they usually hit the poor first and worst. We have known this for a while. The German pathologist Rudolf Virchow described this link between poverty and vulnerability to outbreaks in his 1848 study of a typhus epidemic in Upper Silesia:

"Pandemics and the Poor," by Ben Oppenheim and Gavin Yamey, The Brookings Institution (Books), June 19, 2017. Reprinted by permission.

For there can now no longer be any doubt that such an epidemic dissemination of typhus had only been possible under the wretched conditions of life that poverty and lack of culture had created in Upper Silesia.

What we have not known, until recently, is how best to help the poor protect themselves from pandemics.

To understand why the poor are more vulnerable to epidemics and pandemics and what protections are required, we need to consider how outbreaks first start, how they spread, and how they affect individuals and societies.

Recently, we've been studying pandemics—outbreaks that spread across international boundaries, potentially wreaking enormous health, social, and economic damage. Pandemics are becoming more frequent, not less: Emily Chan and colleagues have shown that the likelihood of pandemics has risen over the last century due to environmental, ecological, and social factors.

How Pandemics Start—and Why They Smolder and Spread

Most pandemics begin with a pathogen leaping from wild or domesticated animals to humans, what is called a "zoonotic spark."

Kate Jones and colleagues have found high levels of spark risk in West and Central Africa, and South and Southeast Asia. These regions are experiencing rapid expansions in human settlements, intensifying agricultural and livestock production, and increasing exploitation of natural resources. Such factors drive contact between humans and animals, amplifying pandemic risks. These regions are also home to most of the global poor.

The first line of defense against pandemics is surveillance: monitoring human and animal populations to spot outbreaks and contain them quickly.

Despite growing international attention, disease surveillance remains weakest in impoverished countries at greatest risk. Such countries are short on labs, infrastructure, and trained epidemiologists. Underinvestment in preparedness reflects the painful choice facing poor countries with high disease burdens: attend to *today's* health burdens or to the potentially far-off (yet inevitable) risk of a pandemic.

These weaknesses mean that in poor countries, isolated outbreaks are likely to go undetected longer and, thus, to smolder and spread.

How They Impact Health—and the Pocketbooks of the Poor

Regardless of where a pandemic starts, once underway, the poor tend to bear the brunt. Low- and middle-income countries (LMICs) have weaker health systems and limited capacity to handle surges in cases. Christopher Murray and colleagues estimate that if a flu pandemic similar in severity to the 1918 Spanish flu pandemic were to hit today, there could be 62 million deaths, of which 96 percent would be in LMICs.

We can curtail pandemics if we quickly develop vaccines and make them widely accessible. However, without vigorous efforts to secure equitable access, vaccine distribution will follow the logic of the market. During the 2009 swine flu pandemic, wealthy countries secured large advance orders for vaccines, but, despite the efforts of the World Health Organization to negotiate donations, poor countries were crowded out—receiving vaccines more slowly than rich countries and unable to cover as many of their citizens.

These same distributional inequalities are also likely to play out within poor countries. The poorest regions in a country are often the most vulnerable since they have fewer pandemic response resources—fewer health workers and clinics and less medicine. When outbreaks begin, the poor are also more likely to have already been suffering from malnutrition and immunosuppressive conditions, which can increase susceptibility to infectious diseases.

Epidemics and pandemics can cause enormous economic damage as workers fall sick, fearful people avoid markets and public places, and quarantines and disease control measures reduce travel and clamp down on trade. Acute economic disruption carries particular risks for poor households, whose livelihoods are already precarious.

All three countries affected by the 2014 West African Ebola epidemic suffered large GDP growth shocks, totaling $2.8 billion in lost GDP. This figure probably underestimates the true economic impact. Victoria Fan and colleagues calculated the "inclusive" cost of outbreaks (the sum of the cost in lost income and a dollar valuation of the cost of early death) and found that for Ebola, the inclusive costs are two to three times the income loss.

Protecting the Poor—a Four-Point Plan for Pandemics

Since poor populations face a higher spark risk—a greater chance that an outbreak will spread in these communities—and a higher likelihood of health and economic shocks, pandemic preparedness efforts must preferentially target the poor. This means doing at least four key pro-poor things:

1. *Focus on countries with high disease burdens and high spark risk.* This requires domestic and international investments in basic public health systems, including investments in human and animal surveillance, paying close attention to addressing vulnerability in the poorest regions within LMICs. We agree with the International Working Group on Financing Pandemic Preparedness that development partners should strengthen financing of national preparedness efforts in LMICs, focusing on "(i) in-country capital investments and one-off spends; (ii) multi-country regional initiatives; and (iii) failed and fragile states where domestic resourcing is not a realistic option."

2. *Track progress in pandemic preparedness.* Governments should be held accountable for improving their preparedness—especially for providing equal protection to all citizens, whether rich or poor. In a recent article, we recommend ongoing monitoring, external evaluations, and the use of pandemic risk and preparedness indices.

3. *Ensure equitable access to pandemic vaccines and medicines.* Strategies could include pre-purchase agreements that specify minimum coverage for poor countries and an equivalent pace of disbursement of these technologies.

4. *Invest now for economic recovery from pandemics.* This requires special facilities, such as the World Bank's Pandemic Financing Facility. In the midst of a severe pandemic, even wealthy countries can face domestic political pressures to spend at home and to clamp down on discretionary aid spending. There is also a role for targeted assistance to poor households through safety nets, cash transfers, or other forms of assistance.

14

Better Tools and Systems Are Needed for Pandemic Preparedness

Bill Gates

Bill Gates is the cofounder of Microsoft and a major philanthropist. The Bill and Melinda Gates Foundation is a nonprofit organization that advocates for global public health and funds charities and scientific research.

While many advances—such as antibiotics, vaccines, and diagnostics—have been made to eradicate major infectious diseases, important gaps still remain that prevent adequate preparation for the next pandemic. The 2014 Ebola outbreak served as a wake-up call. Since then, public and private partnerships have been working toward funding initiatives to develop a comprehensive pandemic preparedness and response system. To prevent future pandemics, we have to prepare just as the military prepares for war. When the COVID-19 virus spread around the world, many saw Gates's remarks as prophetic.

Four years ago, the world was stunned by the Ebola outbreak in West Africa. Panic broke out all over the globe. Governments scrambled to contain the infection. By the time the last patient tested negative for the disease, the outbreak claimed thousands of lives and caused billions of dollars in economic losses.

"The Next Epidemic Is Coming. Here's How We Can Make Sure We're Ready," by Bill Gates, the Gates Notes LLC, April 27, 2018. © 2018 The Gates Notes, LLC. Reprinted with permission.

The 2014 Ebola outbreak was a stark reminder of how vulnerable our society is to epidemics of infectious diseases. We weren't ready then, and we're still not ready now—but we can be. We don't know when the next epidemic will strike, but I believe we can protect ourselves if we invest in better tools, a more effective early detection system, and a more robust global response system.

When the Massachusetts Medical Society asked me to deliver this year's Shattuck Lecture, I knew I wanted to talk about epidemic preparedness. I was honored to address their annual meeting earlier today. Here is the full text of my prepared remarks:

Remarks as delivered
Shattuck Lecture
April 27, 2018
Boston, MA

Bill Gates:

Thank you, Dr. Drazen, for that kind introduction. It's an honor to be invited to deliver the Shattuck Lecture.

Most of the speeches I give on global health are about the incredible progress and exciting new tools that are helping the world reduce child mortality and tackle infectious diseases. Thanks to better immunization and other interventions, child mortality has been reduced by more than 50 percent since 1990. We are on the verge of eradicating polio. HIV is no longer a certain death sentence. And half the world is now malaria-free.

So usually, I'm the super-optimist, pointing out that life keeps getting better for most people in the world.

There is one area, though, where the world isn't making much progress, and that's pandemic preparedness. This should concern us all, because if history has taught us anything, it's that there will be another deadly global pandemic.

We can't predict when. But given the continual emergence of new pathogens, the increasing risk of a bioterror attack, and how connected our world is through air travel, there is a significant probability of a large and lethal, modern-day pandemic occurring in our lifetimes.

Watching Hollywood thrillers, you'd think the world was pretty good at protecting the public from deadly microorganisms. We like to believe that somewhere out there, there is a team ready to spring into action—equipped with the latest and best technologies.

Government agents like Jack Bauer in *24*. Harvard professors like Robert Langdon in *Inferno*. And WHO epidemiologists like Dr. Leonora Orantes in *Contagion*—who even risked getting kidnapped as she pursued "Patient Zero."

In the real world, though, the health infrastructure we have for normal times breaks down very rapidly during major infectious disease outbreaks. This is especially true in poor countries. But even in the US, our response to a pandemic or widespread bioterror attack would be insufficient.

Several things in the last decade have made me pay closer attention to the risk of future pandemics. One was the outbreak of Swine Flu in 2009. While H1N1 wasn't as lethal as people initially feared, it showed our inability to track the spread of disease and develop new tools for public health emergencies.

The Ebola epidemic in West Africa four years ago was another wake-up call. As confirmed cases climbed, the death toll mounted, and local health systems collapsed. Again, the world was much too slow to respond.

And, as biological weapons of mass destruction become easier to create in the lab, there is an increasing risk of a bioterror attack.

What the world needs—and what our safety, if not survival, demands—is a coordinated global approach. Specifically, we need better tools, an early detection system, and a global response system.

Today, I'd like to speak with you about some of the advances in tools—vaccines, drugs, and diagnostics—that make me optimistic we can get a leg up on the next pandemic. And I'll talk about some of the gaps we must address in preparedness and response.

Interestingly, the first Shattuck Lecture—given back in 1890—focused on a pandemic... the Russian flu that struck Massachusetts the previous year. The Russian flu was not especially deadly. But it was the first flu pandemic to spread across continents connected by rail travel—and between continents connected by fast ocean liners. The virus circled the globe in just four months.

But the world was soon in for much worse. Less than 30 years later, the Boston area was one of the first places in the US to feel the deadly effects of the 1918 flu. Military personnel getting off and on ships at the Commonwealth Pier—near where we are meeting today—helped carry the pathogen across the US and back to the battlefields of World War I.

The virus took five weeks to spread across the United States and killed 675,000 people.

The death toll was so great that average life expectancy in the US for that period dropped by 12 years.

Worldwide, the 1918 flu killed an estimated 50 million people, perhaps more.

We have better tools today than we did a century ago. We have a seasonal flu vaccine, although it's not always effective, you have to get one every year, and most people in the world never get the shot. We also have antibiotics for secondary infections of bacterial pneumonia.

Despite these advances, the simulation by the Institute for Disease Modeling shows what would happen if a highly contagious and lethal airborne pathogen—like the 1918 flu—were to occur today.

Nearly 33 million people worldwide would die in just six months.

That's the sobering news. The good news is that scientific advances and growing interest on the federal level, in the private sector, and among philanthropic funders makes development of a universal flu vaccine more feasible now than 10 or 20 years ago.

Our foundation is involved in a variety of research partnerships, including a collaboration between the Icahn School of Medicine at Mount Sinai, GlaxoSmithKline, and PATH.

Their work focuses on several vaccine candidates that did well in animal trials and which are now in human trials.

We are also supporting efforts by others, including the National Institute of Allergy and Infectious Diseases, whose vaccine candidate is expected to advance to human safety trials in about a year.

To broaden efforts even further, today we are launching a $12 million Grand Challenge in partnership with the Page family to accelerate the development of a universal flu vaccine. The goal is to encourage bold thinking by the world's best scientists across disciplines, including those new to the field.

Lucy and Larry Page are also supporting efforts by the Sabin Vaccine Institute to encourage innovative approaches that eliminate the threat of a deadly flu pandemic.

However, the next threat may not be a flu at all. More than likely, it will be an unknown pathogen that we see for the first time during an outbreak, as was the case with SARS, MERS, and other recently-discovered infectious diseases.

The world took an important step last year to begin addressing this risk with the launch of a public-private partnership called the Coalition for Epidemic Preparedness Innovations (CEPI).

With funding commitments of more than $630 million, CEPI's first order of business is advancing the development of vaccines for three of the priority diseases on the WHO list for public health R&D: Lassa fever, Nipah virus, and Middle East Respiratory Syndrome.

CEPI is also working on rapid-response platforms to produce safe, effective vaccines for a range of infectious diseases—almost as quickly as new threats emerge. Later this year, CEPI will announce grants to several companies working with a variety of technologies—including nucleic acid vaccines, viral vectors, and other innovative approaches. The goal is to be able to develop, test, and release new vaccines in a matter of weeks or months, rather than years.

I'm a big fan of vaccines, but they may not be the answer when we have to respond immediately to rapidly spreading infectious disease pandemics. Not only do vaccines take time to develop and deploy; they also take at least a couple of weeks after the vaccination to generate protective immunity. So, we need to invest in other approaches like antiviral drugs and antibody therapies that can be stockpiled or rapidly manufactured to stop the spread of pandemic diseases or treat people who have been exposed.

Earlier this year, the Shionogi pharmaceutical company received approval in Japan for a new influenza anti-viral, Xofluza This single-dose drug stops flu in its tracks by inhibiting an enzyme that the virus needs to multiply.

And PrEP Biopharm, a development stage biopharmaceutical company, has demonstrated in human challenge studies that pre-activating the innate immune response through intranasal delivery of a double-stranded viral RNA "mimic" can prevent both influenza and rhinovirus.

Since the host's innate immune response is non-virus specific, such an approach has the potential to offer protection against other types of respiratory viruses as well.

Monoclonal antibody therapies have also made incredible advances in the last couple of decades, leading to several products for cancer and autoimmune diseases. During the Ebola outbreak in West Africa several years ago, researchers were able to identify and test a promising combination of monoclonal antibodies to treat infected patients.

And a growing pipeline of broadly neutralizing antibodies are being discovered in some individuals exposed to infectious diseases. For example, a small percentage of people infected with HIV develop antibodies with high potency and breadth of coverage sufficient to protect against many strains of the virus. The same is true for some people infected with the flu.

Different sets or cocktails of these exceptional antibodies may protect against a pandemic strain of a virus even if it has genetically evolved. It is conceivable that we could create libraries of these antibodies, produce manufacturable seed stocks, and have them ready for immediate use in an outbreak—or ready to scale up manufacturing if a pandemic ensues. If we can learn how to use RNA or DNA gene delivery effectively, we may not need to make the antibodies at all.

Rapid diagnosis is also critical, especially at the beginning of an outbreak when quarantine, treatment, and other public health measures are most effective. To that end, researchers at the Broad Institute and at UC-Berkeley have developed a highly-sensitive point-of-care diagnostic test that harnesses the powerful genetic engineering technology known as CRISPR.

But instead of using CRISPR to edit DNA, they have programmed an associated protein called Cas13 to hunt for specific pieces of RNA. When Cas13 locates the relevant genetic sequence, it releases a signal molecule that indicates the presence or absence of the target.

In a paper published yesterday in the journal *Science*, the researchers highlighted the field-use potential of this new diagnostic. Using paper strips similar to a pregnancy test—and with minimal sample processing—the diagnostic can check a patient's blood, saliva, or urine for evidence of a pathogen.

What's more, it can test for multiple pathogens at once. It could, for example, identify if someone is infected with Zika or dengue virus, which have similar symptoms.

There are also some interesting advances that leverage the power of computing to help predict where pandemics are likely to emerge and model different approaches to preventing or containing them.

Over the last few years, researchers at the Institute for Health Metrics and Evaluation at the University of Washington have developed a sophisticated computer model that combines data from dozens of sources with geospatial mapping to predict the pandemic risk of infectious diseases.

They recently looked at the pandemic potential of four viral hemorrhagic fevers in Africa—including Ebola. Their analysis confirmed that Guéckédou prefecture in Guinea—where the West African Ebola outbreak originated—was indeed one of the most likely places where an individual Ebola case could lead to a widespread epidemic.

The research also pinpointed dozens of other African communities that are at high risk of outbreaks of hemorrhagic fevers.

Meanwhile, researchers at the Institute for Disease Modeling are pushing the boundaries of computational epidemiology to provide a deeper understanding of both the spread of infectious diseases and the effectiveness of different control and eradication strategies.

In the effort to eliminate malaria, for example, IDM is combining surveillance data with computational modeling to tailor antimalarial efforts to unique local conditions. They are also using quantitative analysis and modeling to evaluate various control strategies for HIV, TB, and to eradicate polio. This kind of research could provide valuable information to help predict disease transmission and identify prevention measures and intervention tactics for epidemics and pandemics.

At the Munich Security Conference last year, I asked world leaders to imagine that somewhere in the world, there is a weapon that exists—or that could emerge—that is capable of killing millions of people, bringing economies to a standstill, and casting nations into chaos.

If this were a military threat, the response—of course—would be that we should do everything possible to develop countermeasures. In the case of biological threats, that sense of urgency is lacking.

The world needs to prepare for pandemics the way the military prepares for war. This includes simulations and other preparedness exercises so we can better understand how diseases will spread and how to deal with things like quarantine and communications to minimize panic.

We need better coordination with military forces to ensure we can draw on their mobilization capacity to transport people, equipment, and supplies on a mass scale.

We need a reserve corps of trained personnel and volunteers, ready to go at a moment's notice. And we need manufacturing and indemnification agreements in place with pharmaceutical companies—with expedited review processes for government approval of new treatments.

Last month, Congress directed the administration to come up with a comprehensive plan to strengthen global health security—here and abroad. This could be an important first step if the White House and Congress use the opportunity to articulate and embrace a leadership role for the US in global health security.

No other country has the depth of scientific or technical expertise that we do—drawing on the resources of institutions like the NIH, the CDC, and advanced research organizations like DARPA and BARDA.

Our biopharmaceutical industry is the global leader in biomedical innovation. And, on the world stage, the US is an influential member of international forums like the UN, the WHO, the G7, and the G20.

The point is that the US can and should play a leadership role in creating the kind of pandemic preparedness and response system the world needs.

As I said at the start, I'm fundamentally an optimist, and that gives me hope that we can get prepared for the next big pandemic.

The global community eradicated smallpox, a disease that killed an estimated 300 million people in the 20th century alone.

We are on the verge of eradicating polio, a disease that 30 years ago was endemic in 125 countries and that paralyzed or killed 350,000 people a year.

And today, nearly 21 million people are receiving life-saving HIV treatment, thanks primarily to the support of the world community.

America's global HIV initiative, PEPFAR, was the catalyst for world action on the AIDS crisis. It's an example of the kind of leadership we need from the US on a broader effort to make the world safer from other infectious disease threats. With strong bipartisan support, PEPFAR has saved millions of lives and shown that national governments can work together to address pandemics.

Somewhere in the history of these collective efforts is a roadmap to create a comprehensive pandemic preparedness and response system.

We must find it and follow it because lives—in numbers too great to comprehend—depend on it.

Thank you for the opportunity to address you today.

15

Lessons from the Ebola Outbreak: Preparation and Surveillance Are Essential

Viroj Wiwanitkit, Ernest Tambo, Emmanuel Chidiebere Ugwu, Jeane Yonkeu Ngogang, and Xiao-Nong Zhou

Viroj Wiwanitkit is affiliated with Surin Rajabhat University in Bangkok, Thailand, and Joseph Ayo Babalola University in Osogbo, Nigeria. Ernest Tambo is based in South Africa and researches biology and health sciences. Emmanuel Chidiebere Ugwu is affiliated with the Department of Human Biochemistry at Nnamdi Azikiwe University in Awka, Nigeria. Jeane Yonkeu Ngogang is on the faculty of biomedical sciences at the University of Yaoundé, Cameroon. Xiao-Nong Zhou is based in Shanghai, China, and works in disease prevention.

The 2014 Ebola outbreak that devastated West Africa made clear the issues related to surveillance and treatment in underserved communities. However, the feasibility of applying the most up-to-date surveillance and containment practices to impoverished countries proves challenging. The authors argue that synchronization among the international research community, the development of diagnostic tools on a local level, and multidisciplinary computational approaches to outbreak prediction and monitoring could prevent future Ebola outbreaks from causing as much devastation as those in the past.

"Are Surveillance Response Systems Enough to Effectively Combat and Contain the Ebola Outbreak?" by Viroj Wiwanitkit, Ernest Tambo, Emmanuel Chidiebere Ugwu, Jeane Yonkeu Ngogang, and Xiao-Nong Zhou, BioMed Central Ltd., January 9, 2015. https://idpjournal.biomedcentral.com/articles/10.1186/2049-9957-4-7. Licensed under CC BY 4.0 International.

The epidemic of the Ebola virus disease (EVD) in West Africa in 2014 continues to present a global concern due to its extremely high mortality potential, and short- and long-term regional and international consequences. The West African EVD outbreak has received much attention from researchers, humanitarian organizations, and international agencies, as well as from public health workers and communities.[1, 2] An article entitled "Need of surveillance response systems to combat Ebola outbreaks and other emerging infectious diseases in African countries," published in the journal *Infectious Diseases of Poverty* in August 2014,[3] concluded that implementation of an effective surveillance response system with early warning alert mechanisms and the ability to measure transmission dynamics is essential to monitor disease epidemics, and consequently prevent and combat this outbreak and the future emerging epidemic. The article also discussed that an Ebola immunization program and travel medicine initiatives are needed. Issues regarding the limitation of the passive surveillance system have been raised by Viroj Wiwanitkit in this letter to the editor, who emphasizes the need for an active disease detection system such as massive population screening and other interventions. This idea has been agreed upon by Ernest Tambo et al. There have also been discussions between Wiwanitkit and Tambo et al. in this letter to the editor on the extreme resource limitations in outbreak areas. Maximizing the contemporary scientific and technological benefits can greatly improve and strengthen the availability of and accessibility to the much-needed tools and systems, including early detection, early warning alert, planning, and emergency responses.

This was further echoed by Professor Wiwanitkit, in this letter on the previous publication by Tambo et al.,[3] who outlined the research priorities for the development of an appropriate combined disease monitoring system along with good policy to allocate the most effective available tools, and enhance technology and information communication in resource-limited settings in different epidemic scenarios. The journal's editor (Professor Xiao-Nong Zhou) thus combined all of these discussions in one paper, in order to further promote research on moving from a passive surveillance system to an active and integrated surveillance response system that will combat and contain the present extending and future outbreak. This article looks at the importance and limitations of each system and calls for the need to foster more research and set priorities aimed towards novel comprehensive integrated surveillance response systems. These systems should be able to collate effective and reliable data that can support evidence-based decisions and policy and guide emergency responses, in addition to serving as early warning and prompt response systems in the prevention, control, and containment of Ebola and future emerging diseases.

Combating Ebola Outbreaks: Other Options Besides Surveillance Response Systems

Viroj Wiwanitkit believes that Ebola outbreaks can be combated by other means besides surveillance response systems. He quotes what Tambo et al. reported in the aforementioned article: "Understanding the unending risks of transmission dynamics and resurgence is essential in implementing rapid effective response interventions tailored to specific local settings and contexts."[3]

The emerging Ebola virus is a serious regional and international consideration with short- and long-term crisis ramifications and consequences on the social, health, and economic statuses of nations. Several attempts have been made to stem out this new emerging viral infection since the first outbreak occurred, however, the control and containment of the disease in West Africa has not been successful. A major concern is its high mortality rate and fate of survivors, especially the thousands of orphans who have been abandoned, as well as the compounded issue of years of political unrest that has been worsened by the Ebola crisis. Up to date, more than 450 health workers have contacted the virus from patients, with over 150 deaths reported.[4] To successfully control the Ebola outbreak, surveillance response systems are undoubtedly important tools. However, whether they are effective enough on their own is questionable. There is a vital need to enhance and strengthen community health education and promotion, local capacity building, and knowledge of EVD and other epidemics, and implement safety measures for vulnerable communities.

In fact, to successfully control and contain the outbreak, urgent and early emergency response preparedness and planning is required. Raabea and Borcherta noted that "effective identification and isolation of cases, timely contact tracing and monitoring, proper usage of personal protection gear by health workers, and safely conducted burials" are essential for success.[5] Surveillance response systems, which are generally used for the management of an outbreak, can be useful, however, they are a passive method as they simply gather data about an already existing infection. Although new computational technology might be applied to predict possible new foci of disease, it is not an actual finding but a computational prediction. Additional active method should be applied to increase the effectiveness of disease control. The use of active disease surveillance such as mass screening is suggested.[6] It should be noted that the asymptomatic Ebola virus infection is possible and might be the reservoir source of infection.[7] Finally, along with standard available techniques, the medical community urgently needs to develop new drugs and vaccines for confronting the possible pandemic of this new emerging disease.

Ebola Spreading in the Poor Settings of West Africa with Inexistent Healthcare Systems

Ernest Tambo, Emmanuel Ugwu, and Jeane Ngogang highlighted that Ebola persistence and spread is due to the poor or inadequate healthcare systems, the impact of mining and conflict events, high levels of illiteracy, and rampant medical, community and environmental capacity building in most of the Ebola affected countries in West Africa, as compared to developed countries. The authors thanked Wiwanitkit for his remarks on how the surveillance and response system to combat the Ebola outbreaks can be improved. As Tambo, who has more than 10 years experience working in West Africa, and his team[8] clearly stated, it is an essential and crucial step to implement surveillance and response preparedness and actions effectively and in a timely manner. Similarly, in other African countries with little passive and periodic surveillance and inherent structural deficiencies, high levels of rural illiteracy and ignorance on epidemics, persistent cultural practices and myths, rumors and the inability of the governments to debunk them, a lack of aggressive public health awareness and community outreach with appropriate health education, fragile healthcare service delivery, maternal-child mortality, slow responses, inappropriate use of protective device and disinfectants, health education media (TV, radio, mobile texts), and limited government funds and reliance on internattional donors such as Global Fund to Fight HIV/AIDS, Tuberculosis and Malaria, it is difficult to contain the spread of Ebola without local surveillance response systems.[8]

Thus, in line with Wiwanitkit's concerns, active and integrated surveillance response systems should be developed with networks of community/environmental workers, which include early warning, early diagnosis, quick reporting, case finding, case tracking and investigation, and prompt appropriate measures including treatment to stop the transmission. In addition, it is also necessary to foster more efforts in new viral diagnostic and drug/vaccine discovery, as well as innovative measures based on local contexts. Tambo et al. also outline that components of new technology development are needed to improve the sensitivity of surveillance response systems.[1] It is clear that inexistent or inadequate healthcare systems and bottlenecks are compounded by other inequalities (majorly illiteracy and multi-dimensional poverty index) in remote African communities and urban settings.[8] It is these local settings with a lack of adequate interventions that play the most important role in the spread of the Ebola virus in the human population.[9] Please refer to Tambo et al's article to understand the current Ebola crisis and what the next steps should be.[1] Tambo et al. will be pleased to work with Wiwanitkit on the topic of proper surveillance response systems design and share lessons and expertise about Ebola and H7N9.

How to Deal with the Problem in Resource-Limited Settings and Future Research Priorities

Wiwanitkit responded that dealing with the problem in resource-limited settings requires local and context evidence in setting health agendas and research priorities. Good planning and effective allocation of resources, which are limited, has to rapidly done.[10] The education of local medical personnel to have the correct knowledge aimed at disease prevention and management is required.[10]

As argued by Tambo et al., the present passive disease surveillance system to combat the Ebola virus epidemic in Africa appears to not be sufficient as the infection is spreading rapidly. In addition, the available disease surveillance systems in many African countries might not be fully effective.[1] Theoretical political commitment, fancy health investment, and human resource development are the major obstacles in building reliable health systems and surveillance responses for disease outbreaks in the region. What is also of interest is that although the disease has been continuously spreading, there are only a few available data on clinical features and epidemiological information.[10] Limited publications are available on these issues.[11, 12]

An extreme limitation of resources is a basic fact for most infectious diseases' endemicity and epidemicity in Africa. The problem of disease control in this continent is related to poverty.[13] The present Ebola virus crisis is the greatest challenge to local disease surveillance and control agencies.[14] As noted by Smith et al., "more support needs to be given to core coordinating capacity in resource-poor contexts."[15] Grants from many countries around the world to combat the problem are a good sign of collaboration. Without a doubt, research and development of new technologies to manage the problem is also useful. As noted by Tambo et al., "improving the sensitivity of the surveillance response system" might be another practical approach for the present crisis.[8] The development of appropriate combined disease monitoring systems, incorporating both passive and active approaches, might be the answer for managing the rapid expansion of the infection. Electronic integrated systems should also be considered and implemented.[16]

Finally, the local national and regional public health policy seems to be an important determinant. A good policy that allocates the available tools and technologies in resource-limited settings in the epidemic scenario is required. The recent international meeting of the relevant West African health ministers to talk about the Ebola crisis is a good sign and gives hope for successful epidemic control.[11] The following research priorities are put forward to respond to the Ebola outbreaks in Africa:

1. Political research to find ways for a synchronized international collaboration to combat the outbreak;

2. Local development of diagnostic tools to help active case search; and

3. Development of a multidisciplinary computational approach/system and a geographic information system (GIS)-based prediction model for closed, up-to-date outbreak monitoring.

References

1. Chan M: Ebola virus disease in West Africa–no early end to the outbreak. *N Engl J Med* 2014,371(13):1183–5. 10.1056/NEJMp1409859

2. WHO Ebola Response Team: Ebola virus disease in West Africa–the first 9 months of the epidemic and forward projections. *N Engl J Med* 2014,371(16):1481–95.

3. Tambo E, Ugwu EC, Ngogang JY: Need of surveillance response systems to combat Ebola outbreaks and other emerging infectious diseases in African countries. *Infect Dis Poverty* 2014, 3:29. 10.1186/2049-9957-3-29

4. Duffin C: Ebola death toll rises in Africa with at least 14 nurses among the dead. *Nurs Stand* 2014,28(50):9. 10.7748/ns.28.50.9.s7

5. Raabea VN, Borcherta M: Infection control during filoviral hemorrhagic fever outbreaks. *J Glob Infect Dis* 2012,4(1):69–74. 10.4103/0974-777X.93765

6. Parkes-Ratanshi R, Elbireer A, Mbambu B, Mayanja F, Coutinho A, Merry C: Ebola outbreak response; experience and development of screening tools for viral haemorrhagic fever (VHF) in a HIV center of excellence near to VHF epicentres. *PLoS One* 2014,9(7):e100333. 10.1371/journal.pone.0100333

7. Leroy EM, Baize S, Debre P, Lansoud-Soukate J, Mavoungou E: Early immune responses accompanying human asymptomatic Ebola infections. *Clin Exp Immunol* 2001,124(3):453–60. 10.1046/j.1365-2249.2001.01517.x

8. Tambo E, Ai L, Zhou X, Chen JH, Hu W, Bergquist R, *et al*.: Surveillance-response systems: the key to elimination of tropical diseases. *Infect Dis Poverty* 2014, 3:17. 10.1186/2049-9957-3-17

9. Bühler S, Roddy P, Nolte E, Borchert M: Clinical documentation and data transfer from Ebola and Marburg virus disease wards in outbreak settings: health care workers' experiences and preferences. *Viruses* 2014,6(2):927–37. 10.3390/v6020927

10. Wiwanitkit V: New emerging West Africa Ebola 2014: the present global threaten. *Asian Pac J Trop Biomed* 2014,4(Suppl 2):S539–40.

11. Baize S, Pannetier D, Oestereich L, Rieger T, Koivogui L, Magassouba N, *et al*.: Emergence of Zaire Ebola virus disease in guinea—preliminary report. *N Engl J Med* 2014,371(15):1418–25. 10.1056/NEJMoa1404505

12. Callaway E: Ebola outbreak tests local surveillance. *Nature* 2012,488(7411):265–6. 10.1038/488265a

13. Xia S, Allotey P, Reidpath DD, Yang P, Sheng HF, Zhou XN: Combating infectious diseases of poverty: a year on. *Infect Dis Poverty* 2013, 2:27. 10.1186/2049-9957-2-27

14. Smith J, Taylor EM, Kingsley P: One world–One health and neglected zoonotic disease: elimination, emergence and emergency in Uganda. *Soc Sci Med* 2014. pii:S0277–9536(14)00412–2. doi:10.1016/j.socscimed.2014.06.044. [Epub ahead of print]

15. Wahl TG, Burdakov AV, Oukharov AO, Zhilokov AK: Electronic integrated disease surveillance system and pathogen asset control system. *Onderstepoort J Vet Res* 2012,79(2):455.

16. Gulland A: Health ministers in West Africa hold crisis talks on Ebola virus.*BMJ* 2014, 348:g4478.

16

COVID-19 Vaccine Development Occurred with Astonishing Speed

David Pride

David Pride is associate director of microbiology at the University of California, San Diego.

If most vaccines take an average of 10 to 15 years to develop and the previous record was four years, then how did scientists come up with several vaccines to protect against COVID-19 in less than a year? This prodigious achievement is a result of advanced technology known as next generation sequencing, which allowed scientists to determine the genetic sequence of the virus that causes COVID-19 immediately. So extraordinary is the science behind the vaccines and treatments for COVID-19 that it's easy to forget how little was known about the novel virus in the early days of the pandemic.

SARS-CoV-2, the virus that causes the respiratory illness COVID-19, has killed approximately 2.2% of those worldwide who are known to have contracted it. But the situation could be a lot worse without modern medicine and science.

The last such global scourge was the influenza pandemic of 1918, which is estimated to have killed 50 million people at a time when there was no internet or easy access to long-distance telephones to disseminate information. Science was limited, which made it difficult to identify the cause and initiate vaccine development. The world is 100% more prepared for the current pandemic than it was 100 years ago. However, it has still affected our lives profoundly.

I am a physician scientist who specializes in the study of viruses and runs a microbiology laboratory that tests for SARS-CoV-2 infections. I've seen firsthand patients with severe COVID-19 illness and have dedicated myself to developing diagnostics for this disease. It's a remarkable testament to science that a novel disease-causing virus has been discovered, the genetic material completely decoded, new therapies created to fight it and multiple safe and effective vaccines developed all within the span of a year—an accomplishment that the journal *Science* has pegged the breakthrough of 2020.

Most vaccines take 10-15 years to develop. Until now the fastest vaccine developed was against the mumps virus, which took four years. Now, in the midst of the SARS-CoV-2 pandemic, one vaccine is already authorized for use in the US, with a second close behind. Other vaccines have already been rolled out in countries across the globe.

Science Fast-Tracked

This pandemic put science front and center. One of the most significant scientific advances in the past 15 years has been the ability to read the genetic instructions—or genome—that encode viruses. The process of sequencing the genome of a virus is called next generation sequencing, and it has revolutionized science by allowing researchers to rapidly decode the genome of a virus or bacterium, quickly and cost-effectively. This strategy was used to determine the sequence of SARS-CoV-2 early in January 2020 before epidemiologists even recognized that it had already spread around the world. Obtaining the sequence allowed for the rapid development of diagnostics for SARS-CoV-2 and to figure out who was infected and how the virus might spread.

SARS-CoV coronavirus was responsible for an outbreak that spanned 2002–2004, but was not particularly contagious and was limited mostly to Southeast Asia.

SARS-CoV-2 has evolved two separate qualities that allow it to spread more easily. First, it has an enormous potential for triggering asymptomatic infections, in which the virus infects carriers who don't experience symptoms and may never know they are infected and transmitting the virus to others.

Second, it can spread via aerosolized particles. Most of these viruses spread via large respiratory droplets, which are visible and fall out of the air within three to six feet. But SARS-CoV-2 can also spread through airborne transmission via much smaller particles that remain in the air for several hours.

While in 1918 people went on blind faith that masking reduced transmission, this time around, science provided us with concrete answers. There have been several studies demonstrating the efficacy of masking. These types of studies inform the public that mask-wearing, social distancing, hand-washing and limiting crowd sizes decrease circulating virus and thus reduce hospitalizations and death. While they don't get much fanfare, these studies are among the most important discoveries in response to this pandemic.

Science Aids Diagnostics

Many tests for the virus are performed using PCR, which is short for polymerase chain reaction. This method uses specialized proteins and virus-matching DNA sequences called primers to create more copies of the virus. These additional copies allow PCR machines to detect the presence of the virus; doctors can then tell you if you are infected. Because of the availability of the virus's genome sequence, any researcher can design primers that match the virus to develop a diagnostic test.

Early on, the World Health Organization developed a PCR test to detect the virus and disseminated instructions on how to use it to researchers and physicians around the globe.

This was a remarkable achievement that allowed countries across the world to rapidly develop diagnostic tests using this template. This distribution changed the course of the pandemic in many countries.

Treatments Have Lowered Mortality Rates

Treatments for infectious diseases often evolve over time. There is no vaccine yet for hepatitis C, but over recent years treatments have evolved from those that make you very ill to those that are highly efficacious with few side effects.

We are now seeing similar things in the SARS-CoV-2 pandemic, just on an accelerated timeline. With the aid of clinical studies, we now have treatments such as steroids, antiviral medications like Remdesivir and infusions of antibodies. Physicians also know how to alter a patient's position in ways that increase the chance of survival.

Vaccine Development Could End Pandemic

This pandemic could end if the virus swept through the population killing millions but leaving the survivors with natural immunity. More likely the virus will snuff itself out when most of the population has been vaccinated with a SARS-CoV-2 vaccine. That is especially true in parts of the world where frequent testing and public health strategies are difficult to implement.

It took many years to develop an influenza vaccine, with the first available in 1942. Other successes with smallpox and polio, and more recent ones like HPV and *Haemophilus influenzae* Type b, have provided blueprints for vaccine development.

Governments across the world have partnered with private companies to expedite the development of SARS-CoV-2 vaccines. This has led to multiple different companies developing their own different versions of vaccines. Normally, these take years to develop; however, by leveraging recent successes and accumulated knowledge, the timeline was accelerated significantly. Normally, new vaccines go through phase 1 (safety), phase 2 (efficacy) and phase 3 (comparison) trials, but as demonstrated in the current trials, phases 2 and 3 can be combined for expediency. And large-scale manufacturing can begin when the vaccine is still in trials, potentially cutting years off the timeline.

Technology is at the forefront of the development of these vaccines. Some of the coronavirus vaccines take advantage of mRNA technology, which essentially programs our cells to develop immune responses against SARS-CoV-2.

Others use viruses as delivery mechanisms for SARS-CoV-2 proteins to which your body develops an immune response. Both types have thus far been shown to be effective, but long-term safety will remain controversial when vaccines are developed on such an expedited timeline.

Lessons Learned

This disease, which began in Wuhan, Hubei Province, China, and was first diagnosed in either November or December of 2019, is the perfect illustration of just how rapidly viruses spread in a connected world. We got previews of what could happen from the recent outbreaks of Ebola and Zika virus, but the spread of SARS-CoV-2 has been on a different level. It has underscored that when we receive warnings about contagious viruses, rapid and decisive action must be taken in all parts of the world to reduce its spread.

Where there is more strict compliance with public health policies, there have been profound reductions in virus transmission.

While the research that has made all this possible might fly under the radar right now, history will record this time as one of the greatest periods for scientific advancements.

17

Total Vaccination Coverage Needs to Be the Goal

Marcel Salathé

Marcel Salathé is an assistant professor of biology and adjunct faculty of computer science and engineering at Pennsylvania State University.

Despite the fact that measles was considered eliminated in the United States as of 2000, recent outbreaks indicate that this is not entirely true. Outbreaks of diseases like measles occur when not enough people are vaccinated against them, and the concept of "herd immunity" helps explain what percentage of the population needs to be immunized in order to prevent an ongoing chain of disease transmission. This lesson has been applied more urgently to the COVID-19 pandemic. Herd immunity for measles requires 90–95 percent of the entire population to be immunized, and since some people are not eligible for vaccination, this means that everyone who can be vaccinated, should be.

The measles outbreak traced back to Disneyland has spread to eight states, with as many as 95 cases reported by January 28. Media outlets are highlighting the rise of anti-vaccination sentiments. Scientists are expressing their dismay at people who reject sound medical advice and put their families and communities in harm's way.

"Herd Immunity and Measles: Why We Should Aim for 100% Vaccination Coverage," by Marcel Salathé, the Conversation, February 2, 2015, https://theconversation.com /herd-immunity-and-measles-why-we-should-aim-for-100-vaccination-coverage-36868. Licensed under CC BY-ND 4.0.

Measles was considered eliminated in the United States in 2000. But if the first month of 2015 is any indication, this year will easily beat the record number of measles cases recorded in 2014.

The narrative during this outbreak, or any measles outbreak really, is that measles is a highly transmissible disease. So transmissible in fact that 90–95% of people must be vaccinated in order to protect the entire population, or achieve what is called herd immunity.

That is partly true. Measles is highly transmissible, not least because people can be contagious days before symptoms develop. But there are three problems with this line of reasoning about vaccination rates.

First, the numbers are based on calculations that assume a world of random mixing. Second, the vaccination coverage is not a perfect measure of immunity in the population. Third, and most problematic in my view, it gives people a seemingly scientific justification for not getting vaccinated—after all, if not everyone needs to get vaccinated in order to attain herd immunity, can it really be so bad if I opt out of it?

What Exactly Is Herd Immunity?

Let's look at the concept of herd immunity first. The basic idea is that a group (the "herd") can avoid exposure to a disease by ensuring that enough people are immune so that no sustained chains of transmission can be established. This protects an entire population, especially those who are too young or too sick to be vaccinated. But how many people need to be immune to achieve this?

In order to calculate the number of people who need to be immune for herd immunity to be effective, we need to know how many people will get infected, on average, by an infectious person.

Imagine that a newly infected person will on average pass on the disease to two other people. Those two will each infect another two people, who will themselves pass it on, and so on, resulting in the classical pattern of an exponentially growing outbreak.

In order to stop the growth in the number of transmissions, we need to ensure that each individual case causes, on average, less than one new infection. So, let's say that one case leads on average to two more infections, but instead we want that number to be less than one. That means at least 50% of the population needs to be immune, so that at most, only one of the two people who might have been infected by an individual will be.

How Many People Need to Be Vaccinated to Achieve Herd Immunity?

So, how do we calculate what fraction of a population needs to be immune to reach herd immunity? First, we need to know what the reproduction number, or R, is. That's how many new cases a single case of an infection will cause.

Imagine that you are infected in a completely susceptible population, and you pass on the infection to five other people (ie $R=5$). In order to prevent an outbreak, at least four out of those five people, or 80% of the population in general, should be immune. Put differently, 20% of the population may remain individually susceptible, but the population would still remain protected.

So if you can estimate the reproduction number for a given disease, you can calculate the fraction of the population that needs to be immune in order to attain herd immunity.

For influenza and Ebola, the number R is about two. For polio and smallpox, it is around five to eight. But for measles it is much higher, somewhere between 10 and 20. And because of that, the goal for measles vaccination coverage is typically around 90–95% of a population.

But there's a problem with this calculation.

The Population Is Not Random

The assumption underlying the calculation for herd immunity is that people are mixing randomly, and that vaccination is distributed equally among the population. But that is not true. As the Disneyland measles outbreak has demonstrated, there are communities whose members are much more likely to refuse vaccination than others.

Geographically, vaccination coverage is highly variable on the level of states, counties, and even schools. We're fairly certain that opinions and sentiments about vaccination can spread in communities, which may in turn lead to polarized communities with respect to vaccination.

And media messages, especially from social media, may make the problem worse. When we analyzed data from Twitter about sentiments on the influenza H1N1 vaccine during the swine flu pandemic in 2009, we found that negative sentiments were more contagious than positive sentiments, and that positive messages may even have back-fired, triggering more negative responses.

And in measles outbreak after measles outbreak, we find that the vast majority of cases occurred in communities that had vaccination coverages that were way below average.

The sad truth is this: as long as there are communities that harbor strong negative views about vaccination, there will be outbreaks of vaccine-preventable diseases in those communities. These outbreaks will happen even if the population as a whole has achieved the vaccination coverage considered sufficient for herd immunity.

If negative vaccination sentiments become more popular in the rest of the population as well, we may start to see more sustained transmission chains. Once those chains are sufficiently frequent to connect under-vaccinated communities, we may again be in a situation of endemic measles.

The solution often proposed is that we should do a better job of convincing people that vaccines are safe. I'm all for it. But I would also suggest that we should stop basing our vaccination policies on models that made sense in a world of constrained vaccine supply, and aim for 100% vaccination coverage among those who can get vaccinated.

This would also solve another problem, often glanced over: There are many people who cannot get vaccinated for medical reasons, either because they are too young, or because they have other conditions that prevent them from acquiring immunity through vaccination.

Herd immunity against measles requires that 90–95% of the *entire* population are immune, whereas vaccination coverage is measured as the percentage vaccinated of the *target* population—which only includes people who are eligible for vaccination. This means that to achieve 95% immunity in the population for measles, vaccination coverage needs to be higher than 95%. This is the scientific argument for a public health policy that aims at 100% vaccination coverage.

More importantly, there is an ethical argument to be made for the goal of 100% vaccination coverage. It sends the right message. Everyone who can get vaccinated, should get vaccinated—not only to protect themselves, but to protect those who can't, through herd immunity.

Organizations to Contact

The editors have compiled the following list of organizations concerned with the issues debated in this book. The descriptions are derived from materials provided by the organizations. All have publications or information available for interested readers. The list was compiled on the date of publication of the present volume; the information provided here may change. Be aware that many organizations take several weeks or longer to respond to inquiries, so allow as much time as possible.

Centers for Disease Control and Prevention (CDC)

1600 Clifton Road
Atlanta, GA 30329
phone: (800) 232-4636
website: www.cdc.gov

The Centers for Disease Control and Prevention is one of the divisions of the US Department of Health and Human Services. Among its many roles is to detect and respond to health threats; promote healthy behaviors, communities, and environments; and put science and advanced technology into action to prevent disease.

Coalition for Epidemic Preparedness Innovation

1901 Pennsylvania Avenue NW
Suite 1003
Washington, DC 20006
website: www.cepi.net

The Coalition for Epidemic Preparedness Innovation was founded in 2017 by the governments of Norway and India, the Bill and Melinda Gates Foundation, the World Economic Forum, and other groups. It is an international partnership to develop and distribute vaccines that can stop future epidemics.

Doctors Without Borders

40 Rector Street, 16th Floor
New York, NY 10006
phone: (212) 679-6800
website: www.doctorswithoutborders.org

Doctors Without Borders is a private, impartial international organization comprising medical experts and other professionals who provide the best medical assistance possible to those in need. It was founded in 1971.

European Centre for Disease Prevention and Control

Gustav III:s Boulevard 40
169 73 Solna
Sweden
website: www.ecdc.europa.eu/en/home

The European Centre for Disease Prevention and Control is an agency of the European Union. Its goal is to strengthen Europe's ability to fight against infectious diseases. Its activities include monitoring, research, response, preparedness, public health training, and health communication.

National Institutes of Health (NIH)

9000 Rockville Pike
Bethesda, MD 20892
phone: (301) 496-4000
website: www.nih.gov/

The National Institutes of Health is a division of the US Department of Health and Human Services. It is America's national medical research agency working to prevent diseases and promote good health.

UNAIDS
Avenue Appia 20
CH-1211 Geneva
Switzerland
phone: +41 22 791 36 66
email: communications@unaids.org
website: www.unaids.org/en

UNAIDS is a jointly sponsored initiative between the United Nations and civil organizations to bring an end to AIDS around the world by 2030. It operates in seventy countries.

United Nations Educational, Scientific, and Cultural Organization (UNESCO)
7 Place de Fontenoy
75007 Paris
France
website: www.unesco.org

UNESCO works to strengthen the links between education and health, promoting better health and well-being for all children and young people around the world.

US Department of Homeland Security
2707 Martin Luther King Jr. Avenue SE
Washington, DC 20528-0525
phone: (202) 282-8000
website: www.dhs.gov/

The US Department of Homeland Security has more than 240,000 employees with the mission to safeguard the United States from potential threats. These threats include outbreaks of infectious diseases. The department was founded in 2002.

US Department of Labor—Occupational Safety and Health Administration (OSHA)

200 Constitution Avenue NW
Room Number N3626
Washington, DC 20002
phone: (800) 321-6742
website: www.osha.gov/

The Occupational Safety and Health Administration was created in 1970 to make sure that workplace conditions are safe and healthy. It creates and enforces standards to ensure men and women can work safe from harm of all kinds, including infectious disease.

World Health Organization (WHO)

Avenue Appia 20 CH-1211 Geneva
Switzerland
phone: +41 22-791-21 11
website: www.who.int

The World Health Organization (WHO) was established in 1948 as the international authority on health within the United Nations system. It employs more than 7,000 people from more than 150 countries in offices worldwide to set standards and establish health policies.

Bibliography

Books

Thomas Bollyky. *Plagues and the Paradox of Progress: Why the World Is Getting Healthier in Worrisome Ways.* Cambridge, MA: MIT Press, 2015.

Nancy K. Bristow. *American Pandemic: The Lost Worlds of the 1918 Influenza Epidemic.* New York, NY: Oxford University Press, 2012.

Mark Honigsbaum. *The Pandemic Century: One Hundred Years of Panic, Hysteria, and Hubris.* New York, NY: W. W. Norton, 2019.

Gina Kolata. *Flu: The Story of the Great Influenza Pandemic of 1918 and the Search for the Virus That Caused It.* New York, NY: Touchstone/Simon & Schuster, 1999.

Alexandra M. Levitt. *Deadly Outbreaks: How Medical Detectives Save Lives Threatened by Killer Pandemics, Exotic Viruses, and Drug-Resistant Parasites.* New York, NY: Skyhorse Publishing, 2015.

Evelyn Lord. *The Great Plague: A People's History.* New Haven, CT: Yale University Press, 2014.

Matt McCarthy. *Superbugs: The Race to Stop an Epidemic.* New York, NY: Avery/Penguin Random House, 2019.

Richard Preston. *Crisis in the Red Zone: The Story of the Deadliest Ebola Outbreak in History, and of the Outbreaks to Come.* New York, NY: Random House, 2019.

David Quammen. *The Chimp and the River: How AIDS Emerged from an African Forest.* New York, NY: W. W. Norton, 2015.

David Quammen. *Ebola: The Natural and Human History of a Deadly Virus.* New York, NY: W. W. Norton, 2014.

David Quammen. *Spillover: Animal Infections and the Next Human Pandemic*. New York, NY: W. W. Norton, 2013.

Pardis Sabeti and Lara Salahi. *Outbreak Culture: The Ebola Crisis and the Next Epidemic*. Cambridge, MA: Harvard University Press, 2018.

Sonia Shah. *Pandemic: Tracking Contagions, from Cholera to Ebola and Beyond*. New York, NY: Picador, 2017.

Irwin W. Sherman. *The Power of Plagues*, Second Edition. Washington, DC: ASM Press, 2017.

Irwin W. Sherman. *Twelve Diseases That Changed Our World*. Washington, DC: ASM Press, 2007.

Marc Siegel. COVID: *The Politics of Fear and the Power of Science*. Nashville, TN: Turner Publishing Company, 2020.

Periodicals and Internet Sources

Yvette Brazier, "Everything You Need to Know About Pandemics," *Medical News Today*, May 22, 2018, www .medicalnewstoday.com/articles/148945.php.

Keith Breene, "7 Deadly Diseases the World Has (Almost) Eradicated," World Economic Forum, May 26, 2017, www .weforum.org/agenda/2017/05/7-deadly-diseases-the -world-has-almost-eradicated/.

Centers for Disease Control and Prevention, "Measles Outbreaks and Cases," November 12, 2019, www.cdc.gov /measles/cases-outbreaks.html.

Elizabeth Dias and Ruth Graham, "White Evangelical Resistance Is Obstacle in Vaccination Effort," The New York Times, April 5, 2021, https://www.nytimes.com/2021/04/05 /us/covid-vaccine-evangelicals.html.

Michaeleen Doucleff, "Next Pandemic: Scientists Fear Another Coronavirus Could Jump from Animals to Humans," NPR, March 19, 2021, https://www.npr.org/sections

/goatsandsoda/2021/03/19/979314118/next-pandemic
-scientists-fear-another-coronavirus-could-jump-from
-animals-to-hum.

Matthew M. Kavanaugh, et al., "Ending Pandemics: US Foreign
Policy to Mitigate Today's Major Killers, Tomorrow's
Outbreaks, and the Health Impacts of Climate Change,"
Journal of International Affairs, October 10, 2019, jia.sipa
.columbia.edu/online-articles/ending-pandemics-us
-foreign-policy-mitigate-todays-major-killers-tomorrows
-outbreaks.

Edwin D. Kilbourne, "Influenza Pandemics of the 20th
Century," *Emerging Infectious Diseases*, Centers for Disease
Control and Prevention, January 2006, www.nc.cdc.gov/eid
/article/12/1/05-1254_article.

Emma Lake, "Disease Outbreak: What Is the Difference
Between a Pandemic, an Epidemic and an Endemic?" *Sun*,
October 18, 2019, www.thesun.co.uk/news/4120912
/pandemic-endemic-epidemic-difference/.

Abrahm Lustgarden, "How Climate Change Is Contributing to
Skyrocketing Rates of Infectious Disease," ProPublica, May
7, 2020, https://www.propublica.org/article/climate
-infectious-diseases.

M. Martini, et al., "The Spanish Influenza Pandemic: A Lesson
from History 100 Years After 1918," *Journal of Preventive
Medicine and Hygiene*, March 2019, www.ncbi.nlm.nih.gov
/pmc/articles/PMC6477554/.

Nidal Moukaddam, "Fears, Outbreaks, and Pandemics: Lessons
Learned," *Psychiatric Times*, November 15, 2019, www
.psychiatrictimes.com/anxiety/fears-outbreaks-and
-pandemics-lessons-learned.

Joe Mullings, "Industry Voices—4 Ways Medical Technology
Can Help Prevent the Next Pandemic, and Even Help Fight
This One," Fierce Healthcare, April 27, 2020, https://www

.fiercehealthcare.com/tech/industry-voices-4-ways-medical
-technology-can-help-prevent-next-pandemic-and-maybe
-even-help.

Mike Scott, "Pandemic Impacts Will Last a Decade While
Climate Change Accelerates," Forbes, January 22, 2021,
https://www.forbes.com/sites/mikescott/2021/01/22
/pandemic-impacts-will-last-a-decade-while-climate
-change-accelerates/?sh=400e502e1618.

Meera Senthilingam, "Seven Reasons We're at More Risk Than
Ever of a Global Pandemic," CNN, April 10, 2017, https://
www.cnn.com/2017/04/03/health/pandemic-risk-virus
-bacteria/index.html.

David Sugerman, "Preventing Local Outbreaks from Becoming
Global Pandemics: FETP Enhances Capabilities to Track
Diseases and Stop Them at the Source," Our Global Voices,
Centers for Disease Control and Prevention, April 17, 2017,
blogs.cdc.gov/global/2017/04/17/preventing-local
-outbreaks-from-becoming-global-pandemics/.

Trisha Torrey, "Difference Between an Epidemic and a
Pandemic," Very Well Health, October 23, 2019, www
.verywellhealth.com/difference-between-epidemic-and
-pandemic-2615168.

World Health Organization, "Antibiotic Resistance," February 5,
2018, www.who.int/news-room/fact-sheets/detail
/antibiotic-resistance.

World Health Organization, "Ebola Virus Disease," May 30,
2019, www.who.int/en/news-room/fact-sheets/detail/ebola
-virus-disease.

World Health Organization, "Ebola Virus Disease—Democratic
Republic of the Congo," August 1, 2019, www.who.int/csr
/don/08-august-2019-ebola-drc/en/.

Index